US AND WORLD MEDICAL CARE

US and World Medical Care

Armand A. Lefemine MD

Copyright © 2012 by Armand A. Lefemine MD.

Library of Congress Control Number:		2012909639
ISBN:	Hardcover	978-1-4771-1996-9
	Softcover	978-1-4771-1995-2
	Ebook	978-1-4771-1997-6

All rights reserved. No part of this book may be reproduced or transmitted in any form or by any means, electronic or mechanical, including photocopying, recording, or by any information storage and retrieval system, without permission in writing from the copyright owner.

This book was printed in the United States of America.

To order additional copies of this book, contact:
Xlibris Corporation
1-888-795-4274
www.Xlibris.com
Orders@Xlibris.com

Contents

Introduction 9
Medicare 13
Medicaid 17
Private Insurance 19
Employer Sponsored Health Insurance 21
Small Employer Group Coverage 22
Cost and Administrative Overhead 24
Health Maintenance Organization 25
Managed Care 26
The Uninsured 29
Other Important Insurance Programs 30
Blue Cross and Blue Shield 32
The Affordable Health Care Act 33
Nurses 36
Recruiting Foreign Nurses to US Health Care Facilities 41
Physician Hospitalists 42
Physicians 43
Workforce 46
Hospitalist 49
Nurse Practitioners 53
Physician Assistant 54
Doctor Burnout 56
Malpractice 58
Demographics 60
Quality of Care 61
Medical Schools and Medical Education 66

Payments 69
Growth in Spending.. 72
Telemedicine 74
Physician Income 76
Physicians for a National Health Program 79
The Canadian Health System and Thoughts on Universal Coverage 81
Costs for 2011 85
Corporate Malfeasance.. 86
Where to from Here? Socialized Medicine? Single Payer? 88
The Patient Protection and Afforable Care Act 90
Socialized Medical Care in Other Well Developed Countries 93
Healthcare in the United Kingdom 95
Comments on United Kingdom 98
Health Care in Italy... 99
Health Care in Germany 101
Health Care in France 103
An Overview of the World 109
Health Systems in Some Foreign Countries 116
Healthcare in Belgium 116
Healthcare in Norway 118
Health Care in Sweden 119
Health Care in Poland 121
Healthcare in Russia 122
Health Care in Turkey 124
Health Care in China 125
Health Care in New Zealand 127
Health Care in Australia 129
Health Care in Indonesia 132
Health Care in India 134
Health in Thailand 137
Health Care in Japan 140
Healthcare in Denmark 145

Health in Brazil 147
Health Care in Argentina 150
Healthcare in Chile 152
Healthcare in South Africa 156
Healthcare in Finland 160
Health Care in the Republic of Ireland 165
Healthcare in Algeria 169
Health in Morocco 171
Health Care in Iran 174
Healthcare in Switzerland 179
Comments 182
Facts and Figures Taken from the PNHP +
 (Patient Protection and Affordable Care Act) 188
Individual Health Benefit Accounts 193
Health Care Reimbursement Account 195
Comprhensive Individual Medical Account 196
The Single Payer Approach for Universal Health Care 198
The Taiwan Experience 202
SGR—The Sustainable Growth Rate 204
The Single Payer Plan: A Solution-The Canadian System 206
Alternative Plans: State-Based Single Payer: Vermont Plan 212
The Netherlands Experience with Managed Competition 214
Trends and Reforms in Managed Care and Insurance 216
What About the VA System: A Model for Health Care 220
Drugs and the Drug Companies 222
Research by Physicians for a National Health Program 225
Uninsured and Underinsured in the United States 227
Corporate Money and Care 232
Big Pharma or the Pharmaceutical Industry 235
Hospice, Inc 237
An Overall Look at a Very Complicated Problem 239
Peripheral Items in Medical Care 242

Mental Disorder 242
Dental Care 244
Prostheses 245
Nursing Home... 245
Nursing Homes in United Kingdom.. 247
Medical Products, Research and Development 249
Healthcare Spending and the Healthcare Debate 252
Health Care Payment 254
Private Insurance and Health Care.. 256
Government Programs 258
The Uninsured 260
Healthcare Regulation and Oversight.. 261
Effectiveness Compared to Other Countries 263
Administrative Costs... 265
Coverage.. 266
Mental Health... 268
Medical Underwriting and the Uninsurable.. 269
Demographic... 271
Food and Drug Administration... 272
The Health Care Debate: Can We Afford PPACA 273

INTRODUCTION

Medical care in the United States is a very complex issue because there are so many parts and so many sources of funding as well as a large group of the population, 50 million, that do not have health care coverage.(Includes 9.9 million non-citizens) The government provides health care to over one third of the population under such popular programs as Medicare, Medicaid, Veterans Administration Healthcare, the DOD (military) Tricare system and the Childrens Health Insurance Program. Each of these is directed at a specific group such as the elderly, veterans, military retirees, indigent children and the disabled. Private insurance such as Blue Cross and Blue Shield and a large number of other insurance companies provide financial coverage for health care generally as a benefit of the job though it can be purchased on an individual basis. The cost of private insurance has been escalating. (13 to 17 percent a year) The large group without any insurance or government coverage are dependent on emergency rooms and the charity of physicians and a large number of publically supported hospitals and foundations. More money per person is spent on health care in the USA than in any other country and a greater percentage of the national income is devoted to health care than any other nation. However access, availability and quality may be the subject of some discussion. Access requires cash, insurance, entitlement by a government program, emergency treatment at a hospital facility, and most important the availability of the right doctor or practitioner on a timely basis. For most people the current system works most of the time though it can be very distressing to call a doctors office only to be told that the next opening is months off or to get a bill from the hospital for emergency treatment and radiology exams that can cost thousands. The stress of an emergency or an acute illness at home that requires immediate attention is something that few of us are emotionally prepared for.

The United States has had one of the best if not the best health care system in the world during the past six decades. Some may debate or doubt that assertion with good reason. The USA pays twice as much yet lags behind other wealthy nations in infant mortality and life expectancy. These are hardly the only and best criteria but there is value in viewing progress in medical care and progress in the delivery of medical care in the years since World War Two. One has to admire the scientific and institutional achievements of our society but the other important aspect that we need to evaluate is about the availability of these to the general public. Public Health Policy including disease prevention, vaccination, treatment of communicable disease, clean water supply and collection of data relating to the state of health in the community is outstanding and we will not dwell on these though they are extremely important when evaluating health care on a national or local level. We will look at personal health care from the point of view of access, fairness, cost, quality and the future.

A true global view of our system is very difficult because so many changes have occurred and are occurring not only in the practice of medicine but in education, in nursing, in malpractice insurance, in hospital organization, and in the cost of medical care on a national as well as local level. The reimbursement for fee-for-service physicians by government agencies and insurance companies has been falling during the past few decades due to formulas that change annually with the net effect being a reduction of income for many physicians. This plus an escalation in malpractice insurance plus increase in office overhead leads many physicians to close their office in favor of a salaried job with a hospital or other medical organization. In medical school women already outnumber men with a probable shift in what specialties are chosen for a career. In some schools there is an increased emphasis on producing more primary care physicians. This emphasis may be influential in distracting new graduates from specialties like surgery which is already suffering from a declining interest in its residency programs at least by graduates from US medical schools. There is a projected shortage of nurses as well as physicians as the population grow. This will be discussed under manpower needs. The delivery of medical care to a nation and to the community has undergone a series of changes that underscores a financial as well as a professional evolution. In the early years of the 20th century almost all medical care was on a fee-for-service basis. Doctors maintained their own offices or started clinics. HMOs (health maintenance organizations) and insurance companies added a new a dimension to the delivery of medical care by offering comprehensive health care for a monthly payment. This model is basic to the systems used by Medicare and dozens of insurance companies and by large HMOs such as Kaiser-Permanente in California. Hospitals provided only beds, equipment, operating rooms and nurses. Some clinics became famous as centers of excellence such as the Mayo Clinic and the Cleveland Clinic. Now the University Hospitals compete on the same level of service. Health Maintenance Organizations such as Kaiser Permanente Plan in California added a new and attractive way of doing business offering complete coverage. Medicare and Medicaid changed not only the reimbursement for services but also assumed the decision making process as to what services were allowed and what the fee schedule would be. Many decisions that used to be the prerogative of the physician are now dictated by the insurance companies or the government agency. On the national level the cost of medical care has increased 10-15% a year such that the US spends about 16% of its GDP or about 2 trillion dollars per year. The US government pays for about 45% of health costs compared to about 86% in the UK.

    The high cost of medical care and the relentless rise in insurance premiums brought about demands for cost control. HMOs or Health Maintenance Organizations and Managed Care Organizations became the favored answer for administrators and government agencies. Kaiser Permanente (1) was often cited as an example of controlling cost without affecting delivery of quality medical care. But administrative changes were imposed by necessity by insurance companies. Some drugs were too expensive or experimental, consultations were reduced by not allowing self referral, office visits were limited in time, admission to a hospital or emergency department would require permission, and postoperative stays were strictly limited. Many patients were turned down for insurance for preexisting conditions. Despite expansion of the HMOs costs continued to rise at an unacceptable rate during the 90s for those covered by insurance or HMOs. The national government has also experienced large increases in the cost of Medicare, Medicaid and the VA programs mainly the result of population growth, increase in the number of retirees and an expansion of eligible groups under Medicaid. Statistics indicate that the cost for family coverage has doubled in the past seven years. These stats also reveal that it costs $6100 a year for the individual American and $2500 per individual for health care in other countries. Are we getting more and better care or are we paying more for what we get? The comparisons are with other well developed and industrialized nations such as Canada, England and Japan where health care is provided to everyone. US health care ranked last when compared with six other industrialized nations reported by Naseem Miller of Global Medical News (2010) on measures of quality, efficiency, patient safety, access to care and equity.

MEDICARE

The nearest thing the United States has to socialized medicine or universal health care is Medicare. At the present time it covers only a small segment of the total population (about 1/3) above the age of 62, but it easily serves as a model for government provided medical, surgical and psychiatric care. Medicare and Medicaid (which insures the indigent) were signed into law on July 30 1965. Since then a number of services and benefits have been added such as renal disease, children services, Hospice, mammography and PAP smears. There have been a number of changes in methods of hospital and physician reimbursement. Prospective payment systems have been developed for hospital inpatient services based on diagnosis related groups and for outpatient services and home health agencies. Physician services payments are based on a fee schedule. This fee schedule has been operating under regulatory modifications and the Medicare Prescription Drug, Improvement, and Modernization Act of 2003, PL 108-173 for controlling inflation in Medicare Payments for services. This brings into play the Medicare Economic Index and a prospectively determined "allowable" rate of growth known as the Sustainable Growth Rate (SGR). Annually there is a threatened reduction in the fee schedule relative value units (RVUs) that are used in determining the actual payment amounts. The SGR encompasses a number of factors, including the rate of gross domestic product growth. Each year the comparison between actual and allowed spending extends back to April 1996, so that years in which total spending exceeds the SGR have a negative impact for years to come. Some changes in the formula have been made and some adjustments in the Medicare Economic index (MEI) have been legislated but recent periods of slow growth and unanticipated high rates of growth in Medicare service volume will produce negative fee schedule updates for several years. Congress enacted the Balanced Budget Act of 1997, which significantly reduced Medicare payment for most provider services. The budget environment will probably make it difficult for congress to commit the funding necessary to restructure Medicare's flawed physician payment system. There are concerns that some of the payment increases allocated by the Medicare Modernization Act of 2003 will be rolled back. A look at what surgeons face when billing for services, in addition to what seems to be an annual reduction in payments, might be helpful. The Medicare physician reimbursement formula is composed of five key components. First each code in the Medicare fee schedule is assigned a work relative value unit (RVU) which estimates the time and intensity involved in performing the service. Each code is also assigned a practice expense RVU to account for direct expenses such as equipment and supplies and a portion of indirect expenses such as rent. Each code is also assigned a professional liability insurance RVU. A geographic practice cost index (GPCI) adjustment is made to the work, practice expense, and liability RVUs to account for geographic differences in providing services. After the GPCI adjustments are made the work, practice expense and liability RVUs are added together to arrive at the total RVUs for a specific code. Finally this sum is multiplied by the Medicare conversion factor to determine final payment. If any portion of the formula is reduced total payment for the code is reduced. Each year the Centers for Medicare and Medicaid services (CMS) updates the rates it pays Medicare providers. In order to update the Medicare physician fee schedule CMS updates the conversion factor. This update is determined in part by the sustainable growth rate (SGR) formula. Since 2002 the SGR has yielded a negative update to the conversion factor which means the conversion factor will be decreased instead of increased. In 2002 the conversion factor was cut by 5.2%. Congress took action in 2003, 2004, and 2005 to avert additional cuts to the conversion factor. A cut in 2006 went into effect but was repealed in February when congress passed the deficit Reduction Act of 2006(DRA). This froze the Medicare conversion factor at the 2005 level. Two factors are the primary causes of the conversion factor cuts: increased volume and unfunded pay fixes. If spending for a single year exceeds the expenditure target, physician spending is cut the following year, to recoup the excess cost. For example if the expenditure target for one year is 60 billon dollars and the actual spending is 70 billion dollars, the conversion factor will be cut the next year to make up the 10 billion dollar difference. The goal is to cut the conversion factor enough to bring year two expenditures in at 50 billion dollars. Since 2002 spending on physician services has exceeded the expenditure targets due to an increase in volume and intensity of services. Currently SGR debt is approximately 47 billion dollars. There is a cap on how much the conversion factor can be cut in one year which means that physicians will be paying back the overages until 2015 through a series of yearly cuts to the conversion factor. If not for the cap the conversion factor would be cut 28% in 2008. The SGR formula allows physician spending to grow at the rate of real per capita gross domestic product or approximately 2% per year. However since the year 2000 physician spending has risen approximately 10% per year. Part A spending, or the hospital, grew only an average of 2.7% a year. While most surgical services have a volume growth of 2% or less other physician services such as imaging, office visits, physician-administered drugs, and minor in-office procedures have experienced growth rates of 7-25%. Unfortunately all growth is treated the same and all physicians are cut equally under the SGR. The reason for the volume increases is that Medicare beneficiaries are older and sicker than ever before. Another reason is that many services have moved from the inpatient to the outpatient setting and funding has not been redistributed from Part A to Part B. Advances in technology and drugs have led to greater medical and surgical interventions. Under the policy of "budget neutrality" increases in some services means a decrease in other services. Minor increases in some emphasized services such as primary care can lead to a significant decrease in other specialties such as surgery. Reimbursement for many surgical codes has declined in the past 15 years. While gimmicks such as RVUs and SGR limitations may appeal to a conservative lawmaker there will be significant consequences if reimbursements for services continue to fall. These are all details that physicians of all specialties must contend with or at least be aware of if they are to remain in business and/ or plan for the future. It is one of the reasons that doctors offices have an employee or employees to deal with the complexities of billing and collecting money. It becomes a significant overhead expense. And this part of the billing and collecting probably represents only 30% or 40% of the total because there may be dozens of different private insurance forms to contend with. The business details may require more attention than the specialty these days. The annual drama over possible 11th hour congressional intervention to prevent cuts in payments for service under the sustainable growth rate (SGR) formula continue. Under the final Medicare physician fee schedule for CY 2012 without a congressional change in the controversial sustainable growth rate (SGR) formula payments to physicians will be reduced by 27.4% for services in CY2012 which is less than the 29.5% reduction that CMS had originally estimated. The current political climate in Washington is such that a cut in reimbursement for physicians is a real possibility. All requests to remove the SGR or fix a broken system so far have failed. CMS is required to update the relative work values every five years. A key part of the process is the advice it receives from the American Medical Association's Specialty Society Relative Value Scale Update Committee (RUC). On December 1, 2006, CMS published a Final Rule with Comment Period, which updated relative work values, revised the method for calculating the practice-expense values, and implemented earlier legislative provisions related to payment rates for imaging services. The final rule made substantial changes in relative values for physician work and practice expenses.

Medicare has instituted number of quality regulatory programs that add to an already complicated professional and administrative organization. The CMS continues on its quest to recoup what it believes to be billions of dollars in overpayments made to hospitals. The government continues its attempts to reduce physician payments though these reductions are usually overturned by congress. There is a Recovery Audit Contractor (RAC) program that works to uncover fraudulent activity and recover overpayments to hospitals. CMS claims that there were 10.8 billion dollars in overpayments in 2007 alone. There is The Tax Relief and Healthcare Act signed into law in 2006 which expanded the law which expanded the RAC program nationally to look at medical records. Quality improvement organizations (QIO) focused on one, two, and three day stay and review programs for high risk diagnosis-related groups. Surgical procedures will also be looked at with a critical eye. There is a Medicare Administrative Contractor (MAC) program which coordinates Medicare Part A and Medicare Part B payments under a single processor looking for billing mismatches. Present On Admission (POA) was initiated in 2007 along with severity adjusted DRGs which creates joint liability for both physician and hospital. And then there is Medlearn Matters on Condition Code 44. This is a prior to discharge requirement, which means hospitals and physicians must determine accurate patient status before the patient is discharged. CMS has clearly demonstrated through the RAC program that lack of medical necessity is one of the largest causes for identified and recovered overpayments. Nearly one-third of the identified and recovered overpayments in fiscal year 2007 resulted from this category. There must be documentation using evidence-based and literature-backed documentation to support the patients status. The physicians job has become much more complicated and time consuming and probably more expensive. This does not complete the list of programs and demands on the physician. There is a recently implemented Pay-for-Performance program. There is legislation authorizing payment for physicians who report on quality of care.

MEDICAID

MEDICAID, authorized under title XIX of the Social Security Act, was enacted to provide health care services to low income children deprived of parental support or caretaker relatives, the elderly, the blind and individuals with disabilities. Medicaid is a state run program supported by block grants from the government and a state reimbursement that varies from state to state and at times has been so low as to discourage participation by doctors. Coverage under Medicaid can be spotty because there are 50 state plans financed by a General Fund appropriation and government reimbursement is variable. Medicare financing is from a Medicare Trust Fund which is derived principally from payroll taxes. The CMS or Centers for Medicare and Medicaid is one of the largest purchasers of health care in the world. Medicare increased from 19 million enrollment in 1966 to 42 million in 2005. Medicaid enrollment has increased from 10 million in 1967 to 44.7 million in 2005. The CMS spent approximately 484.3 billion dollars or approximately 20% of federal outlays in 2006. The only agency that spent more of the Federal Budget was the Social Security Administration.

The Centers for Medicare and Medicaid Services has 4750 employees but does most of its work through third parties. It processes over one billion Medicare claims annually; it monitors quality of care; it provides the states with matching funds; and it develops policies and procedures for the best care. CMS also assures the safety and quality of medical facilities; it provides health insurance protection for workers changing jobs and maintains the largest collection of health care data in the United States. Other activities for which CMS is responsible include The State Children's Health Insurance Program, The Clinical Laboratory Improvement Amendments of 1988 (CLIA) and implementation of the insurance reform provisions of the Health Insurance Portability and Accountability Act of 1996 (HIPAA). Based on latest projections Medicare and Medicaid (including state funding) represent 33 cents of every dollar spent on health care in this country. It provides 48 cents of every dollar received by US hospitals and 28 cents of every dollar that is spent on physician services. Fifteen percent went to Managed Care. It is the largest source of payment for health care for persons with Acquired Immune Deficiency Disease (AIDS).

CMS plays a leading role in health care Quality improvement. (3) CMS Quality agenda, set by its Quality Council, has membership from across the agency and is chaired by the administrator. The CMS vision is that health care is safe, timely, effective, patient centered, efficient and equitable all of which correspond to the Institute of Medicine's *Crossing the Quality Chasm report*. At the core of CMSs resources are its quality improvement organizations (QIOs). Congress created the QIO program in 1982 to provide a nationwide network of healthcare organizations to help practitioners and providers improve. QIOs are helping providers move toward public reporting and pay-for-performance quality improvement environment in hospitals, physicians' offices, nursing homes, and home health. Medicaid spending has come under fire on several occasions because of its rapid growth. It covers more than 50 million people.

PRIVATE INSURANCE

Many insurance companies compete for the business of insuring all those not covered by Medicare and Medicaid, the VA, or the military and for the Medigap business that pays for the deductibles and the portions not covered by CMS. Blue Cross and Blue Shield Association is the largest of these with member companies in each state. From small beginnings the BC and BS brands have become the largest health care providers in the country serving more than 94 million people in all regions of the country by 2006. Insurance Premiums have gone up 78% since the year 2000 (13% a year) Wages have gone up only 20% since 2000. Kaiser Family Foundation statistics indicate that more than 155 million Americans get their health insurance through their jobs. Employers on average pick up 84% of the cost for individuals and 73%for families. In Massachusetts health insurance is expected to increase 13% in the year 2007. Overall the average cost of health insurance for the individual is $4,242 a year; for a family the total cost averages $11,480 and higher which represent burdensome expenses for the self-employed and the employer. The rising cost of health care is one reason that employers increasingly find it difficult to offer health insurance as a benefit. Since 2000 the percentage of firms offering health benefits has fallen to 61% from 69%. Census figures show that we added 1.3million people to the ranks of the uninsured in the year 2005. In Massachusetts where health insurance is now mandatory the monthly premiums vary from $625 to $1,763 with the HMOs being the lowest cost and BCBS being the highest cost. But the deductibles are significantly higher for the HMOs. Another nuance pushed by the Bush administration is the high deductable insurance plans and health savings account. They have lower monthly premiums but require consumers to pay more of the initial cost of their health care. Kaiser estimates that about 2.7 million workers are enrolled. In 2007 there were 46 million people in the US (15% of the population) without health insurance for at least part of the year. According to United States census approximately 85% of Americans have health insurance. Nearly 60% obtain it through an employer. Today the number without health insurance is probably higher because many workers who have lost their jobs have also lost their employer-provided health insurance. The percentage of non-elderly population who are uninsured has been generally increasing since year 2000. Private health insurance may be purchased on a group basis (e.g. a firm for employees) or on an individual basis. Most Americans receive their insurance through an employer sponsored program. United States Census Bureau indicates that 60% of Americans are covered through an employer while 9% purchase insurance directly. There is a joint federal/state system for regulating insurance known as the McCarron-Ferguson Act though the federal cedes primary responsibility to the state which may require specific types of care or services. State mandates generally do not apply to health plans offered by large employers due the preemption clause of the Employee Retirement Income Security Act.

Employer Sponsored Health Insurance

Employer sponsored health insurance is paid for in part by the business or firm or government as part of an employee benefit package. Nearly all large employers in America offer group health insurance to their employees. The typical large-employer PPO is typically more generous than Medicare or the Federal Employees Health Benefits Program. Typically employers pay about 85% of the insurance premium for their employees and about 75% of the premium for their employees dependents. The employee pays the remaining fraction of the premium usually with pre-tax/tax-exempt earnings. Health benefits provided by employers are also tax favored or even on a pre-tax basis if the benefits are offered through a section 125 cafeteria plan. The disadvantages relating to employer sponsored insurance are that the employee might be paid less because of expense and loss relating to change of jobs or loss of job. Costs for employer-related health insurance are rising rapidly. Costs for employer-paid health insurance have increased 78% since 2001. Wages have risen 19%, inflation has risen 17% according to a study by the Kaiser Foundation. Average premiums, including both the employer and employee portions were $4704 for single coverage and $12,680 for family coverage in 2008. In 2007 the employee Benefit Research Institute concluded that the availability of employment-based health benefits for active workers in the US is stable though the "take-up rate" has fallen somewhat. Effective January 1, 2014 the Patient Protection and Affordable Care Act will impose a $2000 per employee tax penalty on employers with over 50 employees who do not offer health insurance to their full-time workers. In 2008 over 95% of employers with at least 50 workers offered health insurance. Although large firms are much more likely to offer retiree health benefits than small firms, the percentage of large firms offering these benefits fell from 66% in 1988 to 34% in 2002.

SMALL EMPLOYER GROUP COVERAGE

About 59% of employers at small firms in the US provide employee health insurance The percentage of small firms offering coverage has been dropping since 1999. Small firms that are new are less likely to offer coverage than the ones that have been in existence. Only 24% of those that have been in existence less than 5 years did. Self funded health care (provides health and disability with its own funds) is not a practical option for most small employers. Beneficiary cost sharing is higher among small firms than large firms. Insurance brokers play a significant role in helping small employers find health insurance for a commission ranging up to 8%. Premiums can vary by age and they may also vary by health status. However with the Patient Protection and Affordable Care Act effective, by 2014, all insurers will be fully prohibited from discriminating against or charging higher rates based on pre-existing medical conditions. Individual health insurance is primarily regulated at the state level now before the Patient Protection and Affordable Care Act is activated, consistent with the McCarran-Ferguson Act.

There are many different health insurance policies that are available on a private level in the market place that offer specific types of services or health care but the numbers are small and are not of importance on a national level. State mandates generally do not apply to the health plans offered by large employers due to the preemption clause of the Employee Retirement Income Security Act. Early hospital and medical plans offered by insurance companies paid either a fixed amount for specific diseases or medical procedures or a percentage of the providers fee. The relationship between the patient and the provider was not changed. The patient received medical care and was responsible for paying the provider. If the service was covered by the policy the insurance company was responsible for reimbursing or indemnifying the patient based on the provisions of the insurance company (reimbursement benefits). Health Insurance companies whose services are not based on a network of contracted providers or that base payments on a percentage of provider charges are still described as indemnity or fee-for-service plans. The United Health Group was brought to task because a national billing data base that was in use by health plans to determine reimbursements to those who use out of network physician services because insurers were underpaying for out of network expenses by 10-28%. The billing database which is operated by the United Health Group subsidiary Ingenix Inc, will be replaced with an independent database run by a qualified non-profit organization. This illustrates how databases, fee schedules, and even work ratings and overhead reimbursements have been manipulated by the insurance industry.

Blue Cross and Blue Shield Brands are the oldest and largest of health benefits companies. These companies offer coverage for individuals, families, and groups that include everything from long term care, maternity care, dental, prescription drugs, and occupational and speech therapy, to mental health and wellness. BC was born in 1929 when Justin Ford Kimball offered a way for 1300 school teachers in Dallas to finance 21 days of hospital care by making small monthly payments to the Baylor University Hospital. The Blue Shield concept grew out of the lumber and mining camps of the Pacific Northwest where employers who wanted to provide medical care for their workers made arrangements with physicians who were paid a monthly fee for their services. From these small beginnings the BC and BS brands have become the largest health care providers in America serving more than 94 million people in all regions of the country by 2006. BC and BS have worked closely with labor since the depression and now provide health benefits to more union workers and their families than any other national carrier. Since Congress enacted the Federal Employees Health Benefits Act in 1959, BC and BS have enrolled over 50% of the federal workforce, retirees, and families. Since 1966 when Medicare was launched BC and BS have provided an important infrastructure that has helped move the program forward. The Blue System processes the majority of Medicare claims at a total $163 billion. The Blue System now offers a worldwide medical coverage for expatriate workers in US based companies doing business abroad. One-in-three Americans now have BCBS coverage.

COST AND ADMINISTRATIVE OVERHEAD

A significant perhaps the most significant cost in the American system of medical care is the administrative overhead. The private marketplace has created a massive bureaucracy that dwarfs the size and costs of Medicare. Medicare's overhead averages about 2% a year. In 1995 Medicare reported administrative expenses of 2.9 billion or less than 1% of budget. In a 2002 study for the state of Maine, Mathematica Policy Research Inc. concluded that the administrative costs of private insurers in the state ranged from 12% to more than 30%. And much of the insurers' administration is directed toward denying claims. Billing and paper work consume at least 20% of California's privately insured health spending (estimated at 26 billion dollars). Projected nationally these figures indicate that approximately $230 billion of health spending was devoted to insurance administration in 2005. If one could eliminate the paperwork of billing, marketing and review of claims the estimated savings would be over $160 billion. An analysis by James G Kahn revealed that overall 21% of private health spending went to billing and an additional 13% went to non-billing administrative functions. A 2003 study by Himmelstein and Woolhandler found that healthcare bureaucracy accounted for 31% of US health spending—about 400 billion—versus 16.7% in Canada which has a single payer national health plan

Health Maintenance Organization

A health maintenance organization (HMO) is a type of managed care organization (MCO) that provides a form of health care coverage that is fulfilled through hospital and doctors, and other providers with which the HMO has a contract. The Health Maintenance Organization Act of 1973 required employers with 25 or more employees to offer federally certified HMO options. Unlike traditional indemnity insurance an HMO covers only care rendered by these doctors and other professionals who have agreed to treat patients in accordance with the (HMO) guidelines and restrictions in exchange for a steady stream of customers. Benefits are provided through a network of providers. Providers may be employees of the HMO (staff model), or employees of a provider group that has contracted with the HMO (group model) or members of an independent practice association (IPA model) HMOs may also use a combination of these approaches (netmodels).

Managed Care

Managed care is used to describe a variety of techniques intended to reduce the cost of health care and improve the quality. (managed care organizations). Many of these techniques were pioneered by HMOs but they are now used in a wide variety of private health insurance programs. Through the 1990s managed care grew from about 25% of employees with employer-sponsored coverage to the vast majority. Many managed care programs are based on a panel or network of contracted health care providers. In addition to the selected healthcare providers, these programs all emphasize preventive care and formal utilization and quality review. Provider networks can be used to reduce costs by negotiating favorable fees from providers and creating financial incentives for providers to practice more efficiently. A survey in 2009 by America's Health Insurance Plans found that patients going to out of network providers are sometimes charged extremely high fees. Gone are the days when you might find that kindly old doctor who might spend some time with you. Network plans may be either closed or open. With a closed network enrollees' expenses are generally covered only when they go to network providers. Only limited services are covered outside the network, only emergency or out of area care. Most HMOs are closed network plans. Open network plans provide some coverage when an enrollee uses a non-network provider but usually at a lower benefit level. Most preferred provider organizations are open-network. Those that are not are often described as exclusive provider organizations or EPOs as are point of service plans (POS). The terms 'open panel' and 'closed panel' are sometimes used to describe which health care providers in a community have the opportunity to participate in a plan. In a closed panel HMO, the network providers are either HMO employees or members of large group practices with which the HMO has a contract. In an open panel plan the HMO or the PPO contracts with independent practitioners providing participation in the network to any provider in the community that meets the plans credential requirements and is willing to accept the terms of the plans contract. There are other managed care techniques that stress: disease management, patient education, wellness incentives etc. Over time the operations of many Blue Cross and Blue Shield operations have become more similar to those of commercial health insurance companies though they continue as insurers of last resort. Historically, commercial insurers, Blue Cross and Blue Shield plans and HMOs might be subject to different regulatory oversight in a state. However today it is common for commercial insurance companies to have HMOs as subsidiaries and for HMOs to have insurers as subsidiaries. At one time the distinctions between traditional indemnity insurance, HMOs, and PPOs were very clear; today it is very difficult to distinguish between the products offered by the various types of organizations operating in the marketplace.

The US health insurance market is highly concentrated as leading insurers have carried out over 400 mergers from the mid-1990s to the mid-2000s. In 2000 the two largest health insurers (Aetna and United Health Group) had total membership of 32 million. By 2006 the top two insurers, WellPoint and United Health had total membership of 67 million. The two companies together had more than 36% of the national market for commercial health insurance. A 2007 AMA study found that in the HMO/PPO market one concern accounted for at least 30% of the market. There are other types of insurer products that are available such as disability income and long-term care that many workers and the elderly find desirable but these are expensive and optional on the national scene.

An alternate approach to address increasing premiums was signed into law by George W Bush in 2003 as part of the Medicare Prescription Drug, Improvement and Modernization Act, which created tax-deductible Health Savings accounts(HSAs). These are untaxed private bank accounts for medical expenses, which can be established by those who already have health insurance. Withdrawals from HSAs can be used for qualified expenses including doctors fees, Medicare Parts A and B, and drugs without being taxed. Consumers wishing to deposit pre-tax funds in an HSA must be enrolled in a high-deductible insurance plan with a number of restrictions on benefit design. Currently the minimum deductible has risen to 1200$ for individuals and 2400$ for families. HSAs enable healthier individuals to pay less for insurance and deposit money for their own future health care, dental and vision expenses. HSAs are only one form of tax-preferred health spending accounts. Others include Flexible Spending Accounts (FSAs), Archer Medical Savings Accounts (MSAs) which have been superseded by the new HSAs and Health Reimbursement Accounts (HRAs). These accounts are most commonly used as part of an employee health package. While there are currently no imposed limits to FSAs legislation currently being reconciled between the House and Senate would impose a cap of 2,500$. While both the House and Senate would adjust the cap to inflation, approximately 7 million Americans who use their FSAs to cover out-of-pocket health care expenses greater than $ 2,500 would be forced to pay higher taxes and health care costs. In 2009, Save Flexible Spending Plans, a national grassroots advocacy organization, was formed to protect against the restricted use of FSAs in health care reform efforts. This was sponsored by the Employers Council on Flexible Compensation (ECFC) dedicated to the maintenance and expansion of the private employee benefits on a tax-advantaged basis. Most FSA participants are middle income Americans earning approximately $55,000 annually. Individuals and families with chronic illnesses typically receive the most benefit from FSAs; even when insured this group incurs annual out-of-pocket expenses averaging $4,398. Approximately 44% of Americans have one or more chronic conditions. Because Limited Medical Benefit Plans pay for routine care and do not pay for catastrophic care they do not provide financial security equivalent to a major medical insurance plan. Another option becoming more popular is the discount medical card. These cards are not insurance policies but provide access to discounts from participating health care providers but have serious potential drawbacks for the consumer.

The Uninsured

Based on the census data of 2007 more than 45 million people in the USA (15%of the population) were without health insurance. The number of uninsured especially in the non-elderly has been increasing and the reality is probably closer to 50 million uninsured in 2011. About 38% of the uninsured live in households with incomes over $50,000 and 9.7 million are non-citizens. It has been estimated that nearly one fifth of the uninsured is able to afford insurance, one-quarter is eligible for public coverage and the remaining 56% need financial assistance (8.9% of all Americans) An estimated 5 million of those without insurance are considered "uninsurable" because of pre-existing conditions. The cost of the uninsured will obviously be born by the taxpayer, charity and perhaps by higher insurance premiums. A 2008 Kaiser report found an increased strain on Medicaid and SCHIP programs because of increased enrollment resulting from the economic downturn, (total increase about $3.4 billion). During the last downturn, the Jobs and Growth Tax Relief Reconciliation Act of 2003 included federal assistance to states that helped to avoid tightening their Medicaid and SCHIP eligibility rules. A study published in the American Journal of Public Health estimated that in 2005 in the United States there were 45,000 deaths associated with lack of health insurance.

OTHER IMPORTANT INSURANCE PROGRAMS

Military Health Systems: Active duty service members as well as retired military and their families are provided health care for a lifetime through two major systems: The Department of Defense Military Health System (MHS) and The Veterans Health Administration. The MHS consists of a direct care network of Military Treatment Facilities and a purchased care network known as TRICARE. The military has worldwide treatment centers for its active duty force and TRICARE for those stationed in the US. The Veterans Administration has medical centers and clinics in all states and several in the more populous states that offer the full spectrum of medical and surgical and psychiatric care even retirement and long-term rehabilitation facilities or locked facilities for those that require that kind of care. Most VA hospitals are located at or near Medical Schools with whom they share faculties and staff and research.

Other facilities and services need to be mentioned for the sake of completeness. The State Children's Health Insurance Program (SCHIP) is a joint state/federal program to provide health insurance to children in families that earn too much money to qualify for Medicaid, yet cannot afford to buy private insurance. The statutory authority for SCHIP is under title XXI of the Social Security Act. SCHIP programs are run by the individual states according to requirements set by the federal Centers for Medicare and Medicaid Services and may be structured as independent programs separate from Medicaid. States receive enhanced federal funds for their SCHIP programs at a rate above the regular Medicaid match. There is also an Indian Health Service that has always been provided by the Public Health Service. State Risk Pools came into being in 1976 to enable individuals who are medically uninsurable through private health insurance to purchase a state-sponsored health insurance plan usually at higher cost. Plans vary greatly from state to state both in costs and benefits and in their methods of funding and operation. They serve a very small portion of the uninsurable market—about 182,000 in the US in 2004 and about 200,000 in 2008. Another type of health care program that was signed into law in 2006 is the Massachusetts Health Reform Law that was signed by Governor Romney. At the time of the reform law the population of the uninsured in the state was just 6.4% compared to 15.8% nationally. The reform expanded coverage with an individual mandate, penalties for employers who do not offer health coverage and an expansion of Medicaid and subsidized insurance for adults with incomes of up to 300% of the federal poverty level. Just 1.9% of residents lacked insurance in 2010. However access to health insurance does not guarantee access to health care. One in five working-age adults say they have trouble finding a doctor who will see them. The Connector, the state's exchange has excelled at enrolling uninsured adults into subsidized care but has failed to attract small businesses and their employees. Costs increases are unsustainable. Spending on MassHealth, the program for the poor rose 40% between 2006 and 2010. The subsidized health program for adults was more expensive than expected—$628million in 2008 and 805million in 2009. This was offset in part by a drop in the number who used to turn up at emergency rooms for treatment but the decline was less dramatic than hoped for. For those who do have insurance average monthly premiums rose by 12% between 2006 and 2008.

BLUE CROSS AND BLUE SHIELD

Blue Cross and Blue Shield Brands are the oldest and largest of health benefits companies. These companies offer coverage for individuals, families, and groups that include everything from long term care, maternity care, dental, prescription drugs, and occupational and speech therapy, to mental health and wellness. BC was born in 1929 when Justin Ford Kimball offered a way for 1300 school teachers in Dallas to finance 21 days of hospital care by making small monthly payments to the Baylor University Hospital. The Blue Shield concept grew out of the lumber and mining camps of the Pacific Northwest where employers who wanted to provide medical care for their workers made arrangements with physicians who were paid a monthly fee for their services. From these small beginnings the BC and BS brands have become the largest health care providers in America serving more than 94 million people in all regions of the country by 2006. BC and BS have worked closely with labor since the depression and now provide health benefits to more union workers and their families than any other national carrier. Since Congress enacted the Federal Employees Health Benefits Act in 1959, BC and BS have enrolled over 50% of the federal workforce, retirees, and families. Since 1966 when Medicare was launched BC and BS have provided an important infrastructure that has helped move the program forward. The Blue System processes the majority of Medicare claims at a total $163 billion. The Blue System now offers a worldwide medical coverage for expatriate workers in US based companies doing business abroad. One-in-three Americans now have BCBS coverage.

The Affordable Health Care Act

The Affordable Health Care for America Act House Bill H.R. 3962 was passed in the House of Representatives in November 2009 by the Democrats and later approved by the Senate. This is a landmark Bill. This expansive and expensive Bill will have the following elements

1. Establishes a mandate to purchase private insurance for most individuals with an income above poverty levels
2. Creates a mechanism to enforce the mandate in a sliding scale tax on those who do not purchase health insurance for most legal United States residents with an income above poverty level
3. Prohibits pre-existing condition exclusions
4. Requires adjusted community rating, guaranteed issue, and guaranteed renewal of individual and small group health insurance that limits age rating variation of premiums to 2:1 (200 percent), prohibits gender and health status rating variation of premiums, allows variation of premiums, allows variation of premiums by geographic area, and family (vs individual) enrollment.
5. Prohibits cancellation of coverage except for evidence of fraud.
6. Limits annual out-of-pocket expenses to $5,000 for an individual and $10,000 for a family.
7. Requires Health and Human Services to create a non-subsidized public health insurance plan with pricing based on private industry averages. Three optional levels of coverage are to be offered by the plan which must set premiums at a level sufficient to fully finance the costs of the health benefits and the administrative costs related to operating the plan.

8. Establishes a Health Insurance Exchange (HIE) within a proposed Health Choices Administration to provide a market place for insurers to sell qualifying plans on a public web site
9. Requires the creation of a risk equalization pool that will allow qualifying plans to minimize the impact of adverse selection of enrollees among the plans.
10. Provides a tax credit for low income individuals and families to help pay insurance premiums
11. Requires employers with payroll costs over $500,000 to provide health insurance that meets the minimum standard of coverage allowed in the HIE.
12. Provides for a tax on employers that do not provide the required health insurance.
13. Provides for a tax on couples with adjusted joint gross income exceeding $350,000(80% of this figure for single people)
14. Reduces Medicare payments to hospitals with excessive readmissions.
15. Further expands Medicaid eligibility and scope of covered preventive services, for lower-income individuals and families.
16. Increases Medicaid payments to physicians for primary care.
17. Provides for a phased-in elimination of the Medicare Part D coverage gap and requires drug manufacturers to discount and/or rebate additional qualifying drugs originally excluded from the plan.
18. Requires the Secretary of Health and Human Services (HHS) to develop quality measures for the delivery of health care services in the United States.
19. Establishes the Health Benefits Advisory Committee chaired by the Surgeon General of the United States.
20. Prioritizes any eventual implementation of best practices in the delivery of health care.
21. Establishes a National Prevention and Wellness Strategy along with appropriations for its trust fund.
22. Outlines Administrative Standards that reduce costs and improve service, including the ability for Administrators to determine an accurate total financial estimate at the point of service as well as enabling real time electronic transfer of funds to take place if possible.
23. Cost and Deficit. It is estimated that this program would cost about $940 billion over 10 years. It would theoretically reduce the deficit by $143 billion over the first 10 years (CBO estimate). Another CBO estimate is that it would reduce the deficit by $1.2 Trillion dollars in the second 10 years.

24. It would expand coverage to 32 million Americans who are currently uninsured
25. It would create Health Insurance Exchanges. The uninsured and self-employed would be able to purchase insurance through state-based exchanges with subsidies available to individuals and families with income between the 133 percent and 400 percent of poverty level. Separate exchanges would be created for small business to purchase coverage—effective 2014. Funding will be available to states to establish exchanges within one year of enactment and until January 1, 2015.
26. Subsidies: Individuals and families who make between 100%-400% of the Federal Poverty Level (FPL) and want to purchase their own health insurance on an exchange are eligible for subsidies. They cannot be eligible for Medicare, Medicaid and cannot be covered by an employer. Eligible buyers receive premium credits and there is a cap for how much they have to contribute to their premiums on a sliding scale.

Federal Poverty Level for family of four is $22, 050

NURSES

Attention to the nursing situation is merited. Certainly nurses are one of the centerpieces of a good and adequate system of medical care. They have always represented the well-trained 24-7 empathetic care-giver. Anyone who has required hospital care in the past, before the recent changes, will probably praise the role of the nurse in their comfort and recovery. This is not to overlook the important role they play in outpatient services. To be sure the Nursing Profession has played an important role in expanding and enlarging the number of job levels and the amount of responsibilities that a nurse can achieve. Fifty years ago nurses graduated from three year training programs with the highly respected RN or Registered Nurse diploma. Most were employed by hospitals to fill needs at all levels where patients were treated. Soon the increasing needs and complexities of patient care stimulated two additional classes of nurses subordinate to the RN, nursing assistants and nurses aides. Soon the 3-year RN program was lengthened and expanded to a four year Bachelor program. Expanded training developed into different and more responsible roles for the degree nurse. The bedside patient-caring nurse who did all things from answering call, delivering medicine and rubbing your back, became the administrator of the unit who was responsible for the necessary paper and record work. Now some become Nurse Practitioners who are able to assist the doctor in office practice or operating room and at times may run a solo practice or even an emergency room. Oncology Nurses assume primary responsibility for chemotherapy programs under the guidance of a physician. Nurses Training has also opened up opportunities in industry such as the pharmaceutical companies, child care, mental care, home care, anesthesia, emergency clinics, Hospice, research, teaching, and government. We have passed through a period when many nurses lost their jobs with the downsizing, left the profession because of unhappiness with the new norms, or have retired because of lack of opportunity. Some changed their workplace or retired because the work was too hard as a result of a shortage of nurses. Much of this downsizing was the result of restrictions and changes in the way medical care was delivered imposed by insurance companies in their zeal to reduce cost. It had a negative effect on patient care and poses a problem for assuring the future supply of nurses.

There is general agreement that there is a shortage of nurses and that there will be a shortage for some time to come. Projections released by the Bureau of Labor Statistics in 2004 listed RNs with the largest projected job growth in the years 2002-2012. In 2002 there were 2.3 million RNs employed and this is expected to rise to 2.9 million by 2012. However with retirement and loss of nurses to other jobs or professions, the replacement requirement would be 1.1 million and we may be looking at a shortage of more than a million nurses by the end of the decade. The aging of the nurse population and a failure of replacement loom as factors in a nursing shortage. Peter Buerhaus of Vanderbilt University predicts a further aging of the RN workforce over the next two decades with an RN population roughly the same size as today and about 20% below projected requirements. Although we have seen overall employment of RNs increase approximately 205,000 since 2001 much of the growth was due to foreign born nurses and older women. Nursing schools need to increase their capacity to educate new RNs and especially to accommodate older nurses. Forty percent of all RNs will be older than age 50 by 2010. Nurses increasingly are facing deteriorating working conditions at the facilities in which they work. According to a 2001 *ANA STAFFING SURVEY* 75% of nurses surveyed feel that the quality of nursing care at the facility in which they work has declined over the past years, while 56% believe that the time available for patient care has decreased. In addition 40% of nurses surveyed said they would not be comfortable having a family member cared for at the facility in which they work. And 54% said they would not recommend the nursing profession to their children. An *ANA HEALTH AND SAFTEY SURVEY* reveals that 88% reported that health and safety concerns influence their decision to remain in nursing. More than 70% said that acute and chronic effects of stress and overwork were among their top health concerns. Back injuries, hepatitis, and safety were cited as important concerns by a majority. Solutions recommended included more pay, a reduced workload by reducing the number of patients each nurse must care for, safer working conditions, and greater autonomy for nursing services in decision making. Nurses are also reporting increasing burnout and job dissatisfaction. One of every five working nurses is considering leaving patient care for reasons other than retirement within the next 5 years according to *"The Nurse shortage: Perspectives from Current Direct Care Nurses and Former Direct Care Nurses"*, a 2001 study commissioned by the Federation of Nurses and Health Professionals. Salary levels have been cited as major reasons for dissatisfaction. Nursing School enrollments have been increasing but many applicants are turned away from baccalaureate programs due primarily to a shortage of nursing educators. A study by Sochalski at the University of Pennsylvania found that an increasing number of new graduates aren't going into nursing at all. More than 4 out every 100 female nurses were not working in nursing after graduation. That number is twice as high for new male graduates.

That nurses are important for good patient care is generally accepted. Studies also point out that they are crucial to the safety of the patient. A study on the nursing shortage by Linda Aiken of the University of Pennsylvania School of Nursing found that an estimated 20,000 people die each year because they have checked into a hospital with overworked nurses. This same study found that Americans scheduled for routine surgeries run a 31% greater risk of dying if they are admitted to a hospital with a severe shortage of nurses. This is approximately a fifth of the estimated 98,000 deaths that occur each year as a result of medical errors. If true and corroborated these are indeed astounding numbers and indicative of a crisis. A survey reported in the New England Journal of Medicine Dec 12, 2002 reveals that more than 1/3 of practicing physicians and 40% of the public say that a family member has experienced a medical error. Shortages of nurses, fatigue and overwork are cited as important causes. The results of these and other surveys have reached the Halls of Congress and The Nurse Reinvestment Act was signed by President Bush providing scholarships, loans and Public Service announcements to promote nursing. There is also proposed legislation that would allow more direct input by nurses into the staffing patterns of hospitals and would strictly limit the practice of forcing nurses to work overtime.

There are encouraging and forward looking signs for nursing however. The recent past has not been good for promoting the field of nursing and for providing adequate staffing on the wards and in the ambulatory clinics. Salaries are not the only criterion if staffing is low and the nurses overworked. Nurses and the doctors should determine if staff levels are adequate not the administrators. The marketplace for well-trained and experienced nurses is very competitive. Salaries at a community level must also be competitive if you are to retain your staff or hire more nurses. Nursing or program directors may be offered $115,000 to $140,000. These should be attractive to those new graduates. A revue of salaries at Cape Cod Healthcare reveals that a clinical or staff nurse is competitive when compared with traditional scales of the recent past. A nurse will be paid $40,000 to $60,000 based on experience and longevity. A head nurse or ward manager can make $60,000 to $80,000 a year. A Supervisor can earn $75,000 to $90,000 a year and the Director of Nursing can earn upwards of $120,000. Nurses are one of the centerpieces of a good and adequate system of medical care. Their role has expanded dramatically in the last 50 years from one of bedside nursing care (formerly 3 year training program) to bachelor, masters and PhD degrees, to increased clinical responsibilities as nurse practitioners, clinical nurse specialists, nurse anesthetists, nurse-midwives, operating room specialists and as managers, teachers and administrators. Most of these require a Masters Degree. This brought about a need for Nursing Assistants and Nurse Aides. Some practice medicine such as dermatology or run an emergency room. Oncology nurses assume primary responsibility for chemotherapy programs. Nurse training has opened up opportunities in industry, child care, mental health, home care (the Visiting Nurse Organization), anesthesia, Hospice, research and government. And there are more, the options are endless: psychiatry, diabetes, geriatrics, pediatrics, holistic (acupuncture), occupational health, radiology, rehabilitation, post-operative care, emergency-care, critical-care, transplant nurses, plastic and reconstructive, telehealth, transport nurses, and even specialists in aids and drug addiction. The Nurse Practitioner replaces the doctor in many offices and clinics and does this in a very responsible way. Registered Nurses constitute the largest healthcare occupation with 2.6 million jobs. About 60% of RN jobs are in Hospitals.

We have passed through a period when many nurses lost their jobs because of downsizing. Now there is agreement that there is a shortage of nurses. Projections released by the Bureau of Labor Statistics in 2004 listed RNs as having the largest projected job growth in the years 2002-2012. Peter Buerhaus predicts a further aging of the RN workforce, with the shortage continuing about 20% below projected requirements. Nurses are facing deteriorating working conditions and many feel that the quality at the facility in which they work has declined. Many have left nursing because of stress and overwork. Back injuries, hepatitis and safety are cited as concerns by a majority. An estimated 20,000 people die each year because they have checked into a hospital with overworked nurses. Working conditions vary greatly from pleasant surroundings and regular hours in schools to nights and weekends in hospitals and emergency facilities. Median annual wages of registered nurses were $62,450. The middle 50% earned between $51,640 and $76,570. The highest 10% earned more than $92,240. A Director of Nursing or a Program Director may earn upward of $120,000 a year.

The Nurse Reinvestment Act was signed by president Bush providing scholarships, loans and public service announcements to promote nursing. There is also proposed legislation that would allow more direct input by nurses into the staffing patterns of hospitals and would strictly limit the practice of forcing nurses to work overtime. The demands of insurance companies and the CME have put a lot of pressure on hospitals to control costs by reducing staffing. This has resulted in closing of wards, more ambulatory surgery, more use of rehab hospitals that require less staff and more home care. This has not been a formula for better care. The decrease in staffing in hospitals has also put more work pressure on the remaining staff. Many nurses have retired or quit jobs because of increased stress and excessive duties. Salaries are not a solution if staffing is low and the nurses are overworked.

Staffing levels in hospitals came up for debate in the Massachusetts Legislature back in 2007 because of the complaint that nurses were being forced to care for too many patients at once. The complaint included charge of increased complications, hospital-acquired infections, preventable medical errors longer hospital stays and readmissions. The Coalition to Protect Massachusetts Patients came up with a solution called The Patient Safety act, House Bill 2059. This bill required the Department of Public Health to develop staffing limits as well as waivers for financially struggling hospitals and recruiting incentives to bring nurses back into the profession. At that time there were 100,000 registered nurses licensed in Massachusetts but only 45,000 actually employed in hospitals and thousands who work only part time because many nurses are burned out because of high patient loads. Legislation represented a true compromise between the nurses and the hospital industry, but the bill eventually failed passage because of the hospital industry.

RECRUITING FOREIGN NURSES TO US HEALTH CARE FACILITIES

During the past 50 years the United States has regularly imported nurses to ease its nursing shortage. Although the proportion of foreign nurses has never exceeded 5% of the US nurse workforce, this now is slowly rising, The Philippines has dominated the nurse migration pipeline to the United States. Until the mid-1980s Filipino nurses represented 75% of all foreign nurses in the US nurse workforce. As the US healthcare facilities struggle to fill current registered nurse staffing vacancies, a more critical nurse undersupply is predicted over the next 20 years. Within the first two decades of the twenty-first century the US is predicted to grow at least 18% and the aging population sixty-five and older will increase three times that rate. It is predicted that the US will have a shortfall of 110,000 nurses extending to 275,000 by 2010. Foreign nurses must supply evidence that they have completed the prescribed amounts of didactic and clinical instruction as "first-level" nurses, defined by the International Council of Nurses.

Physician Hospitalists

There is a continual loss of private practitioners to full time salaried jobs with a hospital or the government where there is no overhead and malpractice insurance is a benefit. The Hospitalists now work fulltime in the hospital either in the emergency room or on the wards caring for patients admitted through the emergency department. Many physicians in private practice can no longer make it because of dwindling reimbursements from government or insurance companies. Medical liability has exploded in the last thirty years both in the number of cases and the size of awards. Premiums have gone as high as 160,000 dollars and more depending on the state and the specialty. Service in the emergency room is plagued by a high incidence of malpractice suites. It is difficult for some EDs (emergency departments) to find coverage in certain specialties because of the malpractice problem. Some trauma centers have closed in Florida, Mississippi, Nevada, Pennsylvania and West Virginia. A shortage of physicians is predicted and could run as high as 85,000 by 2020. International medical graduates now make up 26% of the practicing physicians in the United States and though we now graduate over 17,000 MDs a year there is a need for more medical schools to fill the training slots that that are now going vacant.

PHYSICIANS

As important as nurses are to medical care, physicians are the center post upon which it all hangs. The changes wrought by the insurance and government programs in the last 25 years has perhaps affected them more than any of the players in the drama of caring for the sick, the infirm, and all those who are well or worried and need guidance. In the beginning third party payers were a godsend for many physicians because it meant that many who might not pay or could not pay their bill would pay. Physicians in general have always been regarded as well to do by the general population and the specialists such as surgeons made more money than their general practice counterparts. In truth, incomes varied widely with the type of practice, location, the wealth or poverty of the patients and the altruism of the practitioner. Altruism was a necessary characteristic for survival in most cases. It is probably true that the big city specialist had a large income and it is also true that the small town doctor had to run hard during long days and busy weekends. Many of us were fortunate to have such doctors as friends. How many of us remember the $2 office visit without an appointment or the $5 house call because we could not make it to the office. The rush to specialization almost immobilized the medical profession but general practice was salvaged by many new programs at the medical schools emphasizing general practice as a specialty. The growth of the Blues and other insurance entities plus the introduction of Medicare and Medicaid changed the whole system of payment or reimbursement. The rising costs of medical care in general were associated with an increase in the cost of physician and hospital services. It is true that physician incomes were rising and hospital costs or reimbursement were almost inflationary. This put extraordinary pressure on the insurance companies and other agencies all of whom instituted Caps on what could be charged for services. In addition to the Cap there were additional reductions applied to the Cap when payment was made. These reductions were variable but often amounted to 20-30% of the approved Cap. A familiar scenario in a solo office situation was that 25-30% did not pay bills, the rest depended heavily on their insurance payment and patients rarely responded to supplemental bills. Some insurance policies paid directly to the patient rather than to the doctor and the check was known to finance a vacation rather than pay the surgeon.

Fees for surgery, office visits, office procedures, and hospital care have continued to escalate. But so has the overhead. In order to get a reasonable fee for a service one has to start high and expect a reduction. There is a ying-yang or tit-for-tat game that must be played. It is all very subtle. The overhead of the present day office and practice has increased substantially. In addition to the secretaries who answer the phone and makes appointments and pay the bills and greet the patients there is a need for a full time manager for the myriad of insurance forms, questionnaires, deductibles, supplementary billings, physical exam forms, and financial correspondence in general. A nurse is certainly helpful for preparing the patient but may be a luxury. Many offices use or require a Nurse Practitioner. Office practice in many areas is no longer profitable. There is a continual loss of private practitioners to full time salaried jobs at a hospital or with the government where there is no overhead and malpractice insurance is a benefit. We might say that malpractice insurance has become the albatross of the medical profession. For some unfortunate practitioners it is the black knight that destroyed them. The loss of some surgical specialties such as gynecology in some areas of the country has been devastating. Access to medical and surgical care are dependent on our ability to attract high caliber students to train for the profession and our ability to provide the graduate doctor with the opportunity not only to pursue his specialty but to have an adequate income without the threat of unreasonable liability. We must compete for talent in a world that is willing to pay well for high-grade services. Medical liability has exploded in the last 30 years both in number of cases and size of awards or settlements which are often used as a way of removing the onus of a legal battle without admitting guilt. In the surgical world annual premiums have gone from five or six thousand dollars to as high as $160,000 and more depending on the specialty and the state. Medical liability is a significant contributor to the high cost of medical care and to a decrease in availability of services. Trauma Centers are closing because they are the source of many medical malpractice suits and it has become difficult or impossible to get critical surgical specialists to staff them or to take call. This crisis in care has been commented upon in recent reports by the Institute of Medicine and the American College of Surgeons who report that hospital emergency departments and trauma centers across the country are severely overcrowded, emergency care is fractured, and surgical specialists are often unavailable.

A potential, and in some places, a crisis in patient access to emergency surgical care may illustrate the factors that play in the problem and that must be attended to if we are to solve the problem. The Emergency Department (ED) has become the point of universal access to our health care system. It is also the patients final safety net when sick or injured. It has also highlighted the problems of surgical call, shortage of some surgical specialties, medical liability, and appropriate compensation for the surgeons who provide surgical services. In some specialties the insufficient number of participants in emergency call panels has reached crises proportions. Surveys by some specialty organizations reveal that a majority of surgeons take ED call 5 to 10 days a month. Some more often. Hospital By-Laws often allow older surgeons to "opt out" and they frequently take advantage of this option. Then there is the liability problem.

The high incidence of malpractice suits, lack of reimbursement, and interference with the part of practice that produces the income has caused some surgeons to exhibit market responses to these pressures by restricting practice to a subspecialty or omitting hospital based care altogether making them unavailable for on-call panels. Hospital ED administrators say that these surgeons frequently relocate to ambulatory surgery centers. This puts a tremendous amount of pressure on the system that provides normal emergency care and is the backup in case of a terror attack. Nearly half the EDs were at or beyond capacity in 2005. According to the National Center for Health Statistics there were 114 million ED visits in 2003 and this represents a 26% increase since 1993. Formally designated trauma centers as part of a state or regional trauma care system are known to provide the highest quality care to severely injured patients. A March 2005 Harris Poll revealed that Americans appreciate the importance of receiving treatment at a trauma center in the event of a life threatening injury. Yet in 2002, Health Resources and Services Administration found that only eight states met all the recognized criteria for a fully developed trauma care system although 26 states met most criteria.

Workforce

Staffing all the sources of health care is becoming a problem not only because of the organizational changes wrought by insurance demands, malpractice liabilities, federal rules and burdensome rise in cost each year but also because there are important trends and predicted shortages in the number of people who deliver care and staff all the various offices, hospitals, clinics, emergency rooms, trauma centers, and operating rooms predominantly physicians and nurses.

Workforce shortage especially in surgery is becoming an important problem. The number of surgeons trained each year has remained stable for the past 20 years. Physician work force analysts now project a shortfall in specialties that are crucial to community-based emergency care. US population growth has outpaced the supply of surgical specialties. An analysis by the Lewin Group of the American Hospital Association's ED and Hospital Capacity Survey of 2002 showed that neurosurgeons, orthopedic surgeons, general surgeons and plastic surgeons were among the specialists in short supply for ED on-call panels. A similar survey by the American College of Emergency Physicians in 2005 showed that nearly three-quarters of ED medical directors believe that they have inadequate on-call specialist coverage. The problem of a surgical workforce is compounded by a graying of the workforce and retirements. It is also complicated by the trend for general surgical residents to pursue fellowships and subspecialization that limit their ability to handle the broad range of problems that are encountered in the ER. It has long been recognized that there are very few training positions in neurosurgery, just 130 openings each year. Compare this with 4,700 positions in Internal Medicine. There are about 3200 practicing neurosurgeons in the US and a third of those are older than age 55 which reduces their availability for the call list. It takes approximately 7 years to train a neurosurgeon and the pool of available surgeons is not getting bigger. The inadequate number of specialists for emergency services is taking its toll on quality of care. Some ED administrators have said that lack of specialty coverage poses a significant risk to patients. The rising demand for emergency services and the declining availability of surgical specialists is creating a crisis in prompt access to emergency surgical care.

In 2007 the Society of Thoracic Surgeons reported that many cardiothoracic surgery residency programs did not fill all the training residency slots for the fourth time. Only 61% or 87 of 130 filled by match date. As residency applications decrease the number of practicing cardiothoracic surgeons in the United States is also falling. Applications to cardiothoracic surgery residency programs have dropped 51% from a high of nearly 200 in 1995. The American Medical Association found that the number of active cardiothoracic surgeons decreased between 1995 and 2004. The same report showed growth rates of more than 20% for specialties like plastic surgery and dermatology. The many years of training, lifestyle sacrifices, and declining compensation (nearly 50% decline in Medicare reimbursement for coronary bypass since 1987) have combined to make this part of the profession less attractive to many medical students. Because the specialty takes 12-14 years of training a future shortage of cardiothoracic surgeons is dangerously imminent.

Surgeon recruitment for rural hospitals is already a major problem. A projected shortage of almost 30,000 surgeons over the next 20 years may make things worse. Researchers estimate that 101,838 surgeons will need to be trained by 2030 to address the projected shortage in the US of 29,138 surgeons in surgical specialties: obstetrics and gynecology, orthopedic, general, otolaryngology, urology, neurosurgery and thoracic surgery.

The model used assumes a US population of 364 million by 2030 and it assumes equal population growth in urban and rural areas. The American Hospital association estimates that there are 3012 urban hospitals serving 82% of the population and 1,998 rural hospitals serving 18% or 56 million Americans. Based on these assumptions the total number of surgical hires over the next 19 years will be 83,507 for urban hospitals and 13,953 for rural hospitals This means that urban hospitals must hire 4,175 surgeons per year or 27.7 surgeons per hospital while rural will need to hire 698 surgeons per year or 7 surgeons per hospital. These figures of course are educated guesstimates but it is fact that rural hospitals are already facing a dramatic loss of general surgeons. In rural hospitals general surgery is essential because general surgeons account for 60% of the revenue. What is happening now is that about 34% of general surgeons are notifying their administrators of retiring or leaving in 2 years. Rural hospitals have always had difficulty recruiting and hiring because of professional and social isolation, cross coverage, insufficient training for many of the problems and women's preference for urban areas.

Similar concerns and predictions abound for General Surgery an important and crucial part of general medical and emergency care in all communities rural as well as city. A substantial number of Americans must travel to the next county or beyond to receive necessary or life-saving surgical treatment. A shrinking supply of general surgeons is one of the prominent concerns of the Affordable Care Act with a new payment incentive for surgeons who practice in underserved areas. But this incentive does not address a problem the size of which may actually be a projected shortage of almost 30,000 surgeons over the next 20 years. Researchers reporting in the Thoracic Surgery News (May, 2011) estimate that 101,838 surgeons will need to be trained by 2030 to address a projected shortage in the United States of 29,138 surgeons in seven surgical specialties: obstetrics and gynecology, orthopedic surgery, general surgery, otolaryngology, urology, neurosurgery, and thoracic surgery. The need for such specialists or to put it another way the shortages will be more acute. The model used predicts that population growth will be equal in urban and rural areas. The national Residency Matching Program of 2007 revealed that 22% of general surgery positions were filled by medical graduates who are not from the US, a 5% increase from the previous year. Even in surgical specialties considered to be more competitive such as orthopedics and plastic surgery international medical graduates (IMGs) constitute 6% of the positions filled in each field. In 2006 IMGs composed 15% (8,399 of 55,142) of the fellows of the American College of Surgeons practicing in the United States. The US Medical Licensing Examination and personal attributes are considered adequate for selection rather than where the candidate went to medical school. There is a complicated bureaucratic process that these candidates must endure which in itself selects only those that are committed to receiving a US training.

There is one additional category for physician surgeons that should be mentioned and that is Surgical Assisting. Many surgeons start to think of retirement as they approach the age of 60-year mark. Once the decision to retire is made, retirees need to figure out what they will do with all their spare time. For people used to working 100 hours per week sitting around is not likely to be a viable option. A solution for some surgeons in Canada has been surgical assisting. Some surgeons in the vicinity of Toronto scrub in on daily elective operations. Surgical assisting is supplied 24/7.

HOSPITALIST

We need to mention the Hospitalist as one of the newer trends and methods of approaching medical care and emergency surgical care. The quality of acute surgical care in the US is threatened by a shortage of surgeons performing emergency procedures. And the availabity of physicians on a community level is decreasing because of rising costs of uncompensated service, liability concerns, declining reimbursement, and lifestyle considerations. Doctors are closing their offices and becoming employees of the hospital because of high overhead, and reduced income, that depends on the vagaries of insurance companies and government gyrations when it comes to reimbursement for services. The Hospitalist is nothing more than an MD in the employ of the local hospital to perform his specialty or training according to assignment and need. They are found in the emergency room, on the wards and in the operating rooms. They have all the advantages of salary, benefits, regular hours paid for malpractice insurance and even vacation time. Though most of their work comes through the emergency room the hospital or more likely the Health Care Corporation that runs community clinics where urgent care is provided. John Maa and colleagues report their experience using the Surgical Hospitalist as a model for emergency surgical care because of a shortage of surgeons performing emergency procedures, because of the rising costs of uncompensated care, liability concerns, declining reimbursement and lifestyle considerations. They hypothesized that a surgical hospitalist would improve timeliness of care, ED efficiency, physician satisfaction, resident supervision, continuity of care, and revenue generation. Three surgical Hospitalists cared for 853 patients during one year, ages 17 to100 presenting with abdominal pain (66%), infection(18%), malignancy (6%), hernia (4%), and trauma (3%). Fifty-seven per cent of consults originated from the ED, 8% came from other surgeons. Mean time to consult was 20 minutes. Average waiting time for patients with acute appendicitis to undergo surgery was reduced from 16 hours to 8 hours. Forty-two percent of consults resulted in an operation and revenue increased as the number of billable consults rose by 190%. The private practice of surgery is changing or will change. A survey of ED physicians reported shorter ED times, better patient satisfaction, improved professionalism and resident supervision, and better overall quality of care.

What are some of the underlying reasons why some specialists are opting out of emergency care. Time, money and liability. The single most important factor shaping the surgical workforce is declining reimbursement. Emergency services are frequently uncompensated and on top of that insurance payments for all procedures have been declining for two decades. When you consider that much of this work and call is at night and on weekends with serious interruption of their routine practice and lifestyle, it is understandable that it undermines the surgeons willingness to take call. A recent report from the Center for Studying Health System Change noted that surgical specialists are more likely to provide charity care than are other specialists or even Primary Care physicians probably because of their emergency on-call responsibilities. NTDB data confirms that surgeons bear the significant brunt of uncompensated care provided to severely injured patients. According to data compiled from more than 1.5 million patient records at 565 US trauma centers "self-pay" is the largest single payment category for trauma center patients (21%) followed by Medicare and Medicaid. While hospitals may draw upon special federal and state financing streams to offset the costs of providing care to patients with little or no health insurance coverage, physicians and surgeons do not have such luxury. Furthermore Medicare payments for many operations that elderly patients require are considerably lower than they were in the 1980s and this is without adjustment for inflation between 1989 and 2006. Many private insurance plans and Medicaid use the Medicare fee schedule as the basis for their own payments thus these trends are repeated throughout the health care system. The overall decline in practice income makes it difficult for surgeons who are in solo or small group practice to shoulder the burden of caring for patients who are unable to pay. Information from Centers for Medicare and Medicaid Services indicates that the reimbursement situation will only worsen as the sustainable growth rate system produces further across-the-board payment reductions, amounting to an additional 39% in the next nine years. Medical specialists have used an increase of volume as a way of offsetting a reduction for service reimbursement but this will not work for surgeons. Volume rates for surgical procedures are not growing, in fact for many surgical services volume is shrinking.

Surgeons will of necessity react to these pressures and threats to their livelihood and careers. In some cases surgeons restrict their practices by subspecializing or limiting their practice to ambulatory centers. A recent survey revealed that 38% of neurosurgeons now limit the types of procedures they perform. Of these, 57% have eliminated pediatrics, 13% no longer provide services related to trauma, and 11% no longer perform cranial procedures. Some surgical specialties that require hospital facilities have developed their own specialty facilities equipped to provide only a limited range of non-emergency procedures.

Liability is equally important as a factor affecting the willingness and availability of some specialties for taking emergency room call.(ED). There is a genuine concern that ED patients will sue. Surveys by the American College of Surgeons and the American Association of Neurological Surgeons/Congress of Neurological Surgeons revealed that more than one third of the respondents had been sued by a patient who was first seen in the hospital ED. A 2005 hospital ED administrators survey revealed malpractice concerns as the principal factor discouraging specialists from providing ED coverage. Liability premiums have simply outpaced the payments that they receive for their services to a largely uninsured patient population. Surgeons are even leaving states with the most severe liability problems. In addition to having trouble recruiting surgical specialists the problem has even forced the closure of trauma centers in Florida, Mississippi, Nevada, Pennsylvania and West Virginia. The surgical specialties with the highest malpractice premium increases are the ones most needed for services in Emergency Departments and Trauma Centers.

Another source of discrimination and pressure on physicians and surgeons who provide services in EDs is the denial of payment by insurance companies (Uniform Accident and Sickness Policy Provision Law(Model 180, UPPL) if the insured (patient) is intoxicated or under the influence of any narcotic. Since alcohol is involved in some way in 30% to 50% of all traumatic injuries this has been a major loss of income for those physicians providing emergency treatment. Physicians have even been reluctant to test for alcohol as a factor in the accident because of this provision in the law in 38 states. Most trauma surgeons believe that it is important to identify the problems and provide intervention when needed. In consideration of these facts the National Association of Insurance Commissioners (NAIC) passed a new model law in 2001 which would prohibit insurers from denying coverage at trauma centers on the basis of intoxication. To date only eight states have adopted this model law.

The looming doctor shortage will not be confined to surgeons and emergency room physicians. The number of US medical school students going into primary care has dropped 51% since1997 according to the American Academy of Family Physicians (AAFP). The AAFP is predicting a shortage of 40,000 family physicians in 2020 when the demand is supposed to spike. US health care system has about 100,000 family physicians and will need 139,531 in 10 years. Currently only about half the necessary number needed to meet demand are pursuing this specialty. At the heart of the rising demand will be 78 million Baby Boomers who turn 65 in 2011. Health Care legislation that extends insurance coverage to underserved patients and the 50 million who lack insurance will fuel the demand and the need. This group of primary care-givers which includes family physicians, general internists, and pediatricians will be the gate keepers that keep people out of the emergency rooms with its high costs. Typically older adults seek care from generalists nearly three times a year, double the rate of those under 65. These practitioners will probably be doing more urgent care and less preventive services. This could lead to the development of "medical homes" where teams of physicians, nurse practitioners, physician assistants and others provide primary care. Reimbursement for services may have to be increased to attract more graduates and provide more satisfaction.

Nurse Practitioners

The Nurse Practitioner is an advanced practice registered nurse (APRN) who has completed graduate-level education (either a Masters or a Doctoral level degree) All Nurse Practitioners are registered nurses who have completed extensive additional education, training, and have a dramatically expanded scope of practice over the traditional role of nurse. To become licensed or certified to practice, Nurse Practitioners require certification in an area of specialty (such as family, pediatrics, women's health, adult health, acute care etc) and are licensed or certified through Nursing boards rather than medical boards. The core philosophy is individualized care as well as the effects of illness on the family. NPs also provide guidance on prevention, education, and research. NPs treat both physical and mental problems including prescribing medication and can serve as the primary healthcare provider and see patients of all ages. In the United States, because the profession is regulated by the state the NP may work independently or have a collaborative agreement with a physician for supervision. There has been a gradual transition in the requirements for practice as a nurse practitioner. In the 1980s Nurse Practitioner educational levels required graduate-level masters degree programs. Subsequently the national certifying organizations and state licensing boards began to require a masters degree for NP practice. Once again there are changes in the field, and by 2015 all new NPs will need to be trained at the doctorate level as a Doctor of Nursing Practice. Established NPs will be grandfathered in.

PHYSICIAN ASSISTANT

A Physician Assistant/ Associate (PA) is a healthcare professional trained and licensed to practice medicine with limited supervision by a physician. A Physician Associate/Assistant is concerned with preventing, maintaining, and treating human illness and injury by providing a broad range of health care services that were traditionally performed by a physician or medical practitioner. Physician assistants conduct physical exams, diagnose and treat illnesses, order and interpret tests, counsel on preventive health care, assist in surgery, give medical orders and write prescriptions. They work in hospitals, clinics, and other types of health facilities and exercise autonomy in medical decisions as determined by their supervising physician, surgeon or medical practitioner. The professional requirements typically include at least two years of post-graduate education. The medical model is designed to complement physician training rather than the nursing model as nurse practitioners are. They are not to be confused with medical assistants who perform administrative and simple clinical tasks with limited post secondary education. In the US the profession is represented by the American Academy of Physician Assistants. The PA profession was first proposed in 1961 and the first class of Physician Assistants in 1965 was composed of former US Navy hospital corpsmen. The curriculum was based on the fast track training of medical doctors during World War II. It was not until 1970 that the AMA passed a resolution to develop educational guidelines and certification procedures. As of June 2011 there were 154 accredited PA programs in the United States. The Majority are graduate programs leading to the award of Masters degrees in either Physician Assistant Studies (MPAS), or Medical Science (MMSc) and require a bachelor's degree and GRE or MCAT scores for entry. Most of these are graduate level training. While some are offering a clinical doctorate degree (Doctor of Science Physician Assistant or DScPA) PAs are not required to possess the doctorate to hold license and practice. PA training is usually 2 to 3 years in duration for a total of 4 to 7 years of post secondary education. The didactic training of PA education consists of classroom and laboratory instruction in medical and behavioral science followed by rotations in internal medicine, pediatrics, family medicine, emergency medicine, surgery, obstetrics and gynecology, and geriatric medicine. A graduate from an accredited PA program must pass the NCCPA-administered Physician Assistant National Certifying Exam before becoming a PA-C; this certification is required in all states. In addition, a PA must earn and log 100 continuing Medical Education (CME) hours and re-register his or her certificate with the NCCPA every two years. Every six years a PA must also recertify by successfully completing the Physician Assistant National Recertifying Exam (PANRE). PAs are medical professionals. They obtain medical histories, perform physical examinations, do procedures, order treatments, diagnose illnesses, prescribe medication, order and interpret diagnostic tests, refer patients to specialists, act as first or second assist in surgery. PAs are employed in all areas of medical practice as well as medical administration. And do not necessarily work under a physicians license. PAs in Florida, Kentucky, Puerto Rico and the US Virgin Islands are not allowed to prescribe, order, or dispense, or administer any controlled substance. The PA must have on file a formal relationship with a collaborative physician Supervisor, although he or she may be physically located elsewhere. Veterans Administration is the largest single employer of PAs employing nearly 2000 PAs. According to the AAPA there were an estimated 68,000 PAs in clinical practice as of January 2008. PAs are working in physician offices, prisons, home health care, nursing homes, schools, the VA, counties, and in the federal government as foreign service health practitioners providing care for the state department, the US army and even special forces. As of June 2011 there are 154 accredited PA programs in the United States. It is listed as one of the best jobs in the US based on salary and job prospects. The mean total income for PAs working at least 32 hours per week was $89,987. Physician Assistants working in some specialties such as emergency medicine, dermatology, and surgical subspecialties may earn $100,000-200,000 per year.

Doctor Burnout

There have been a number of articles on the topic of Doctor Burnout. Obviously some specialties are more stressful than others. There are a number of factors that contribute to stress and lack of satisfaction in the job. In addition to the surgeons who are the first to come to mind as susceptible, the internists and primary care physicians are joining the chorus of complaints. Several articles focus on malpractice suits as a cause of psychological distress and career burnout among US surgeons. According to the results published in the November 2011 Journal of the American College of Surgeons malpractice lawsuits against US surgeons occur often and can take a profound personal toll on the surgeon, resulting in emotional exhaustion, stress, and professional dissatisfaction. Malpractice lawsuits were strongly and independently linked to surgeon depression and career burnout. The stress caused by malpractice was rated as equivalent to that of financial worries, pressure to succeed in research, work/home conflicts, and coping with patients' suffering and death. Surgeons who experienced a recent lawsuit reported less career satisfaction and were less likely to recommend a surgical or medical career to their children or others. The surgical specialties reporting the highest rates of malpractice lawsuits in the last 24 months were neurosurgery (31 percent), cardiothoracic surgery (29 per cent), general surgery (28 per cent), and obstetric and gynecologic surgery (28 percent). The lowest rate specialties were otolaryngology (12 percent), ophthalmology (12 per cent), and breast surgery (14 percent). More than 42 % of all US physicians, including surgeons have been sued for malpractice during the course of their careers. In 2008, annual medical liability system costs, including defensive medicine, were estimated at $55.6 billion or 2.4 % of total health care costs. Data from malpractice liability insurers suggest that a majority of malpractice claims are without merit, and nearly two-thirds of claims are dropped, withdrawn, or dismissed. On average the process of claims and litigation takes five years to resolve, ultimately causing a prolonged adverse impact on the physician. Some studies give additional facets of this question of burnout. Burnout is described as a syndrome of emotional exhaustion and depersonalization that leads to decreased effectiveness at work. In the 7900 questionaires that were returned the picture reveals that the responders were in practice 18 years, worked 60 hours a week and were on call 2 nights per week. Overall 40% of responding surgeons were burned out, 30 % screened positive for symptoms of depression and 28% had a mental QOL score >1/2 standard deviation below the population norm. Factors independently associated with burnout included younger age, having children, area of specialization, number of nights on call per week, hours worked per week, and having compensation determined entirely based on billing. Additional data suggests that approximately 1/3 of US surgeons may experience burnout. Younger physicians and female surgeons are at higher risk for burnout than their older colleagues. Additional data suggests that surgeon distress may contribute to their plans to take early retirement. A Canadian survey suggests that on-the-job stress and burnout may be common among Canadian doctors. A 2001 study of rural family physicians found a reported rate of 55%. Another 2008 study of urban family physicians in southwestern Ontario found that 45% had high scores for burnout. While primary care doctors may be especially subject to burnout, the condition can affect any specialty and even interns and residents going through certification. Classic burnout is related to stress brought on by factors such as too much paperwork, long waits for specialists and tests, feeling undervalued, feeling unsupported, difficult patients, and medicolegal problems. It may be expressed as emotional exhaustion, depersonalization, and a low sense of personal accomplishment.

Malpractice

The escalation in the number of lawsuits and the large awards have driven the cost of medical malpractice insurance to celestial heights and this in no small way has contributed to the high cost of medical care in the USA. The effect of malpractice lawsuits on medical care in some areas of the country has been devastating. It has resulted in doctors retiring or relocating, trauma centers closing, obstetrical services disappearing, and doctors avoiding certain procedures for fear of lawsuits. A study by the department of Health and Human Services catalogs some of the impact of excessive litigation. Most cities in Mississippi with a population less than 20,000 no longer have doctors who deliver babies; 44 doctors in Delaware County PA retired or relocated out of state due to rising malpractice insurance premiums; a doctor in a small town in North Carolina decided to retire after his malpractice premium jumped from $7,500 to $37,000; rural West Virginia hospitals have closed their obstetric units because doctors could not afford their malpractice premiums and doctors are reluctant to volunteer at free clinics if they do not have coverage to protect themselves from lawsuits. Malpractice premiums for certain surgical specialties have reached unacceptable and unsustainable heights. Neurosurgery has been known to go well above $100,000 and for obstetrics well above $200,000. The effect of this on the cost to the patient and on third party payers is obvious but the coincidental effects are pressures to practice defensive medicine or surgery and to reduce the scope of practice if it exposes the doctor to high liability activity such as trauma centers or emergency rooms. The indirect cost of defensive medicine that the government must pay is estimated at $24-47 billion per year. Overall lawsuits cost Americans more than $200 billion a year according to Michael Freedman.

A number of states have adopted reforms. In California the annual malpractice premium for an OB/GYN practitioner is $23,000 to $72,000. In Florida, a state plagued by lawsuits, an OB/GYN practitioner pays an annual insurance premium of $143,999 to $203,000. The proportion of OB/GYN practitioners that will have malpractice actions brought against them is 80%. The solution for many is to eliminate obstetrics from their practice. The states have become or will become acutely aware of a healthcare workforce crises due to the skyrocketing costs of professional liability insurance premiums. Nearly one of eleven obstetricians nationwide has stopped delivering babies. In Wheeling WV all the neurosurgeons left town forcing trauma patients to be airlifted to Pittsburgh, PA. Physicians continue to order additional tests due to fear of litigation, many physicians are abandoning high risk procedures. Litigation is out of control, and liability premiums are on the rise. These state governments and physicians were in trouble because of a lack of medical liability reform (MLR). In response to this crisis many states have taken action to defend physicians and their practices through comprehensive medical liability reform (MLR). Medical liability reform was enacted when California passed landmark legislation in 1975. The Medical Injury Compensation Reform Act (MICRA) entitled patients to recover unlimited economic damages, limited non-economic damage awards to $250,000 and placed limits on attorney fees. In the 35 years since MICRA was enacted medical liability premiums increased by more than 1,029% across the country except in California where premiums grew by less than 1/3 that amount largely due to the limits on non-economic damages. These limits have lowered health care costs by an estimated 6 percent saving Californians 6 billion dollars every year on health care. As of 2009 32 states have placed caps on the non-economic damages that a plaintiff can collect from a physician. These caps on non-economic damage as well as on other aspects such as total damage or wrongful death or severe permanent physical impairment have shown that patients have greater access to physicians. For example Texas has seen liability rates cut by an average of 27 per cent as well as a statewide increase in the number of physicians particularly specialists. Stories depicting the toll on medical care by malpractice problems continue to surface and be recorded. In 2002 the trauma center at the University of Nevada Medical Center closed its doors to the public because physicians and surgeons working in the trauma center could no longer afford the costly malpractice insurance premiums arising from the constant threats of lawsuits. With the trauma center closed critically injured patients would have to be transported to a similar center five hours away. It was only after the surgeons agreed to be re-classified as county employees (which provided a shield against excessive lawsuits) that the trauma center reopened its doors. Litigation has become a seemingly unavoidable fact of life for many physicians even if they never committed a negligent act.

Demographics

(AAMC) reveals some interesting demographics that may shape medical care in the future. Of the practicing physicians in the US 27% are female. Of the medical graduates in training programs 42% are women. Specialties with the largest numbers of active physicians remain General Practice, Internal Medicine, and Pediatrics, the specialties that have been most negatively affected by the reimbursement practices of Medicaid and insurance. These are also the specialties with the highest percentage of females as active physicians. In the ACGME resident/fellow trainee group the concentration of females is greatest in Obstetrics/Gynecology and Pediatrics, all considered primary care specialties. These specialties have been adversely affected by medical malpractice suits and by limited reimbursement from Medicare and the insurance companies.

QUALITY OF CARE

The topic of quality in medical care has become prominent in recent years and has been the subject of many statistical reviews. It may be helpful and informative to review a few reports to get a sense for what concerns our health agencies. It is apparent that all is not well in the world of medicine and that efforts to improve quality are called for. A study by the Agency for Healthcare Research and Quality (AHRQ) reported in the Bulletin of the American College of Surgeons (Nov 2005) indicates that patients in hospital intensive care units are at significant risk for preventable adverse events and serious medical errors. The Critical Care Safety Study: *The Incidence and Nature of Adverse Events and Serious Medical Errors in Intensive Care*, shows that more than 20% of the patients admitted to two ICUs at an academic medical center experienced adverse events. Approximately 45% of those events were considered preventable and more than 90% occurred during routine care. CMS (Medicare and Medicaid) has a Quality Council that has emphasized the need for accelerated change and indicated that it will use partnerships, public reporting, pay for performance, quality education and the use of effective health care technologies to promote improvement. At the core of CMS's resources are its Quality Improvement Organizations (QIOs), Medicare contractors that work to improve quality of care. Congress created the QIO program in 1982 to provide a nationwide network of health care organizations to help practitioners and providers improve. QIOs are helping providers move towards a dynamic public reporting and pay-for-performance quality improvement environment in keeping with the Institute of Medicine (IOM's) "Crossing the Quality Chasm" report. QIOs are working with providers in four priority settings: hospitals, physician offices, nursing homes, and home health helping them to eliminate errors and improve quality. This year, CMS and its public-private collaboration with the Hospital Quality Alliance launched a standardized set of hospital quality measures for use in voluntary public reporting. All consumers can access the website "HospitalCompare" for friendly information about the quality of care in the US hospitals. To date more than 90% of approximately 4000 participating hospitals are reporting the 10 clinical starter measures and of those that submitted data 96% are eligible to receive incentive payments. The CMS also added new surgical infection prevention measures and a new pneumonia measure bringing the total number of measures to 20. The two new surgical infection prevention measures are the first of a larger set of patient safety measures that will be collected as part of the Surgical Care Improvement Project (SCIP). The CMS is one of 10 national organizations spearheading this public and private-sector partnership which has the goal of improving patient safety and reducing the incidence of postoperative complications by 25% in US hospitals by the year 2010. In addition the CMS is working through its contractors, with nursing homes, with physician offices using improved information technology and even addressing cultural and racial disparities.

There are other movements afoot to bridge the information gap about quality in medical care. In 1999, the Institute of Medicine issued a report stating that between 44,000 and 98,000 Americans die of preventable medical errors. In January 2004 at a conference in Washington DC that included Majority Leader Bill Frist (R, Tenn) and Senator Hilary Rodham Clinton there was a call for better electronic medical records to help monitor patient care, analyze its effectiveness and disclose that information to consumers. This is a radical departure from traditional medicine which has always treated its review and discussions about deaths and complications as confidential and not for public disclosure. There was a report from the National Committee for Quality Assurance stating that there were 57,000 avoidable deaths each year. Another group the federal Agency for Healthcare Research & Quality reported that quality was subpar in areas such as the treatment of diabetes and cancer detection. Web sites for improving quality and for evaluating care have already multiplied.

The Patient Safety and Quality Improvement Act of 2005 was designed to address these concerns. Under the Act individual and organizational providers can report, discuss and share information on errors and system weaknesses without fear that the information will be used for unintended purposes such as lawsuits. It is estimated that more than half of inpatient deaths are the result of surgical systems issues and more than 70% of surgical adverse events are considered preventable. The PSQIA creates a federal legal infrastructure protecting a provider's "patient safety work product" from non-safety use. To obtain the Law's protections, a provider must assemble patient safety information with a Patient Safety Organization (PSO) in a patient safety evaluation system. This is a complicated way of saying that the gathered information cannot be used to sue the provider.

In March of 2005 after two years of planning, the Brigham and Women's Hospital Center for Surgery and Public Health established a collaboration between Brigham and Women's Hospital, Harvard Medical School and Harvard School of Public Health to investigate quality of care, the availability of adequate surgical manpower and the appropriate use of surgical resources internationally. Research in the Veterans Health Administration (VHA) assessed predictors of surgical outcomes and this catalyzed a movement called the National Surgical Quality Improvement Program (NSQIP) in the United States. NSQIP was instituted in 1994 to collect preoperative, intra-operative, and 30 day outcome variables. With this data the VHA was able to develop risk adjustment models for surgical outcomes and develop best practices. Between 2002 and 2004, 18 private sector hospitals were included in the NSQIP, in a study funded by the Agency for Healthcare Research and Quality (AHRQ). Beginning in 2005 the American College of Surgeons began a private Sector expansion to make the NSQIP available to all surgical practices. The quality improvement program showed impressive results in decreasing morbidity and mortality in the VA system, but implementation in the private sector has been difficult.

In June 2006 the American College of Surgeons NSQIP held its first annual conference to mark the enrollment of its first 100 hospitals and to report the relative performance of the first 37 hospitals. The information presented showed a spectrum of risk adjusted results ranging from good quality, reflected as a low 'observed' to 'expected' ratio (O/E) of mortality or morbidity, to poor quality, reflected as a high O/E ratio of mortality or morbidity. This introduced a kind of transparency not experienced before in medicine or surgery. The Centers for Medicare and Medicaid Services and other government agencies seek to develop accurate and meaningful quality measures and to use this information to reward physicians and other providers who apply evidence-based medicine to improve patient care. In addition to the American College of Surgeons there are a number of consortia that are developing quality measures including the American Medical Association's Physician Consortium for Performance Improvement, the AQA (formerly the Ambulatory Health Quality Alliance), the National Quality Forum, and the Hospital Quality Alliance. The ACS has also formed the Surgical Quality Alliance (SQA) composed of more than 20 surgical specialty societies working together to generate metrics of quality. This certainly represents enormous energy and response to the clamor for transparency and improvement. The college is also developing surgeon researchers to evaluate the massive amount of data that is accumulating. As of 2007, 125 hospitals have been enrolled in NSQIP including two Canadian and one Department of Defense hospital. There is even a Joint Commission Office Based Surgery (OBS) Accreditation

Program created in 2001 as a quality oversight tool for surgical practices with four or fewer practitioners.

This brings us to the most current trend and initiative for quality improvement: pay for performance (P4P). The concept is to reward surgeons for reporting data and good outcomes. Americans could soon be shopping for health care the way they do for other major purchases. Reporting will begin soon and Medicare payments will be reduced for those physicians who do not report. The Society for Thoracic Surgery developed 21 performance measures for adult cardiac surgery from a massive data base of 3 million patients and these have been endorsed by the national Quality Forum (NQF), a quasigovernmental organization that has extensive experience with evidence-based review processes. Third party payers such as CMS and Insurance companies are focusing on possible cost savings. Physicians and other health care providers must keep their focus on quality of care. The CMS has launched the first major evaluation of P4P. The Premier Hospital Quality Incentive Demonstration focuses on 5 surgical procedures or medical conditions for which 34 performance measures are considered. According to the current operational criteria, the top 20% by performance will receive bonuses which by the third year of the program will come from payment reductions assessed to the bottom 20%. During the first year of the CMS demonstration, substantial improvement and savings occurred. As an example, there was a reduction in the frequency of 5 types of complications associated with one of the surgical procedures or medical conditions in one of the states participating in the demonstration project. Extrapolation of that single-state experience to all 50 states results in a potential savings of almost $350 million in one year. If similar reductions are found for the other 4 procedures the savings are huge. Currently the savings are returned to the participating institutions. This model is good for payers but has negative implications for physicians and other health care providers. An alternative approach being considered calls for uniform distribution of savings among all participating providers. P4P is a reality and the medical profession worries that forced participation will be developed further by government and insurance companies.

An article by Jennifer Wilson in the annals of Internal Medicine points to some lessons that foreign medical systems can teach us. US Health Care is among the best in the world but we lag in some areas. Quality is not necessarily tied to cost or the amount of money that is spent. The Health Care Quality Indicator (HCQI) was launched in 2001 and involves 23 participating countries. The Organization for Economic Co-operation and Development (OECD) started this collaboration to measure and compare quality across countries in a meaningful way. While indicators are still being developed current indicators include cancer screening and survival, mortality rates for asthma, heart attack, and stroke; waiting times for hip surgery; and diabetes control and adverse outcomes. The United States has achieved a 5-year breast cancer survival rate that is at least a few percentage points higher than other industrialized countries but lags in its 5-year kidney transplantation survival rate. Many other industrialized countries achieve health care results that are as good or better than the US. For instance the 30 day acute myocardial infarction case-fatality rates are below 7% in Denmark, Iceland and Switzerland compared with almost 15% in the United States. In another example the incidence of major amputations among diabetic patients in Finland, Australia and Canada is less than 10 per 10,000 compared with 56 per 10,000 in the United States. This has produced an intense interest in the electronic medical record (EMR). Industrialized countries vary widely in their acceptance of health information technology such as the EMR. In the US the use of EMR by primary care physicians is just 28%, compared with 79% in Australia, 89% in the United Kingdom, 92% in New Zealand, and 98% in the Netherlands. Use is even higher in Denmark whose national system has nearly 100% participation by primary care providers. The Danish system handles more than 90% of the country's primary sector clinical communications for ordering or obtaining medication data bases, electronic prescriptions, laboratory tests, referrals and to chart consultation notes and hospital discharge summaries. Patients can access their records and check not only their information but also who else has viewed their records. The National Health Service of the United Kingdom is providing all funding for a system that includes creating an electronic care record for all patients, connecting 30,000 General Practitioners to 300 hospitals. This undertaking is estimated to cost about $13 billion but may cost much more. In the United States the cost of a universal EMR would be enormous because of size and the diversity of financing systems. Health systems that have made the transition to EMR are the Department of Veterans Affairs and Kaiser Permanente. Privacy concerns may be a serious impediment. There is no data that EMR reduces cost but it is believed that it improves quality by adherence to guidelines, enhancing disease surveillance and decreasing medication errors.

Medical Schools and Medical Education

There are 125 US accredited medical schools and 17 Canadian accredited medical schools.

The US faced with a new expansive law and a changing landscape of physician and nurse shortages will have to find a way or more likely several ways of increasing workplace manpower. While physicians and Nurses are the basic and authoritative requirements to solving the problems, the solutions will include of necessity all the players of patient care. These will involve Nurse Practitioners (NPs), Physician Assistants (PAs), foreign or International Medical Graduates (IMGs), Foreign trained nurses, Hospitalists (MDs), Residents in training (postgraduate MDs), as well as research or public health MDs. Hospitals, Clinics, Emergency Rooms, Trauma Centers, and private doctor's offices (if any remain), will need to respond to increased demands and pressure. This will all occur in the setting of numerical changes, probably reductions, in the number of certain specialties such as surgery, thoracic surgery, nursing etc. Experts warn that there won't be enough doctors to treat the millions of people newly insured under the law. At current graduation and training rates the nation could face a shortage of as many as 150,000 doctors in the next 15 years, according to the Association of American Medical Colleges. This is predicted in spite of the push by medical schools and training hospitals to increase the number of doctors which now total about 954,000. The greatest demand will be for primary care physicians, such as general practitioners, internists, family physicians, and pediatricians. If there is a shortage it means limited access and longer waiting times. The law does offer sweeteners to encourage people to enter the medical profession and a 10% pay boost for primary-care doctors. A number of new medical schools have opened around the country recently. Four new Medical schools enrolled a total of about 190 students and

12 medical schools have raised the enrollment of first-year students a total of 150 slots according to AAMC. Some 18,000 students entered US medical schools in the fall of 2009. But medical colleges and hospitals warn that there is a shortage of certain medical resident positions. The residency is usually a three or more year period when graduates train in hospitals, clinics or with specialists as Fellows-in-Training usually to qualify for specialty Boards. There are about 110,000 resident positions in the US according to AAMC. Congress imposed a cap on funding for medical residencies. Hospitals rely heavily on Medicare funding to pay for these residency positions which has hurt their ability to expand the numbers of positions. Medicare pays $9.1 billion a year to teaching hospitals for resident salaries, teaching expenses, and operating costs. The new healthcare law will not help the situation. It will probably take 10 years to make a dent in the number of doctors we need. Doctors trained in other countries could help the primary-care situation though there is still the bottleneck with resident slots because they (FMGs) must still complete a US residency in order to get a license to practice medicine independently in the US. As it is some 13% of the available slots are filled by foreign graduates. One provision in the law attempts to address part of the problem. Some residency slots go unfilled each year so the law will pool the funding for unused slots and redistribute it to other institutions with the majority going to primary care and general surgery. Some efforts are being made to interest students and residents in primary care by having them work in satellite clinics. Montefiore Medical center, the university hospital for Albert Einstein College of Medicine has 1220 residency slots. Since 1970 Montefiore has encouraged residents to work a few days a week in community clinics in New York's Bronx section where about 64 Montefiore residents a year care for pregnant women, deliver children and provide vaccines. The debt burdens do influence the choices resident physicians make because some specialties earn more money and carry more prestige.

There is a phenomenon of attrition in surgical residencies. Why this is more common in surgical residency programs is a question that is being investigated because of the decline in interest in General Surgery as a specialty. Dr. Yeo a clinical scholar and a surgical resident noted in her first two years of residency that that they were losing a lot of good people from the surgical residency program. She tried to identify the factors and what the residency was doing wrong. Most years about 1000 surgical residents enter training which means that there are 6000-7000 surgical residents at any one time. One or two of every five surgical residents abandon training, a rate that is much higher than any other specialty that has published their data. Approximately 150 residents leave training programs in any given year and the range of attrition from individual programs ranges from 15% to 33% according to published data. The Surgical Residency Cohort Project funded by the Robert Wood

Foundation seeks to determine the incidence of attrition, the factors associated with attrition, and define possible action that can be taken. Phase one involved in-depth interviews with surgery residents. In initial interviews the most common reasons for leaving surgical training were lifestyle issues (work hours and family life); economic issues and financial compensation. Increased specialization and the fact that other specialties are performing procedures that used to be in the realm of the general surgeon; and personal factors such as the stress involved in taking care of surgical patients. Women leave surgical training at much higher rates than do men. People tend to leave programs after their first year or after their research time and go on to become urologists, anesthesiologists, and psychiatrists. Those that leave after their research time have been in training 4-5 years so that represents a big loss to the profession. Effective intervention measures are still speculative.

PAYMENTS

Payment for services will always be the fundamental problem for the caregivers and those who pay namely the insurance companies and the government agencies particularly Medicare. Fees for services have been on a downward spiral for the past 10 years particularly those of Medicare. This makes salaried positions with large groups, clinics, and government agencies particularly attractive. There is a strong desire and movement on the part of payers to reduce cost and this has been done generally by reducing reimbursements for specific services. Case-in-point would be cardio-thoracic surgery. There has been serious concern about a shortage of surgeons for years. For some reason residencies in cardiothoracic surgery have not been filling or even sought after by our own US graduates. There are many factors at play. One of course is the fact that Cardiology has some very effective techniques for treating acute and chronic problems in coronary disease and another is that reimbursements for surgery (Medicare) have dropped dramatically since 1986. In dollars the reimbursement for a Coronary Artery Bypass has dropped from $4000 to $1500. This is probably not the only factor but it must be remembered that the training of a cardio-thoracic surgeon may involve 8 to 10 years of hard work and little family life. The annual threat by CMS to reduce surgical fees 20% or more is hardly encouraging to the young graduate. It is of interest perhaps to young physicians and even older physicians like myself to see the formula for calculating 2010 physician fee schedule payment. Payment amount is as follows:

2010 Non-Facility Pricing Amount=
(Work RVU*Work GPCI}+
(Transitioned Non-Facility PE RVU * PEGPCI+
{MP RVU * MP GPCI)} * Conversion Factor (CF)

2010 Facility Pricing Amount=
[Work RVU * Work GPCI)+
(Transitioned Facility PE RVU * PE GPCI) +
(MP RVU * MP GPCI)] * CF
The Conversion factor for CY 2010 is $36.0846

To the expert and all those initiated into how you get paid by Medicare these formulae mean something and are important. To the provider of health services these represent only one of the many stumbling blocks that you must learn about in the world of collecting reimbursements from a government agency. Insurance companies have their own forms, all different, that must be complied with in order to receive payment for services. It is no wonder that offices have special employees to handle submissions for payment and fill out the forms. This is not a small expense for the small or independent practitioner. It is also little wonder that many small practitioners are closing their offices and moving on to other forms of practice such as hospitalist or government programs. The development of books of codes of treatments or procedures (ICD-9 and ICD-10) specific for each service has become big business especially for the AMA. These are also subject to frequent changes. There are other possible changes on the horizon that have to do with Medicare patients. The new ICD-10 coding system might seek the ability to privately broker fees with Medicare patients so that Medicare patients could use their benefits to see a physician that does not accept Medicare patients. Another change that is in the Medicare wind is the possibility of bundled payments. Medicare may offer physicians, hospitals and other health care providers the possibility of bundled payments for services. This was mandated under the Affordable Health Care Act. The aim of the program is to incentivize clinicians to work together and provide better continuity of care resulting in better quality and lower costs. The new bundling program offers four ways that health care providers can receive a bundled payment, three of which provide payment retrospectively and one that offers prospective payment. For example, under one retrospective model providers would agree on a target payment amount for the episode of care and providers would be paid under the original Medicare fee-for-service system, but at a negotiated 2% to 3% discount (or greater). At the end of the care episode the total payment would be compared with the target price and providers would be able to share in the savings. The prospective payment model would work differently. Under that option CMS would make a single bundled payment to the hospital to cover all services provided during the inpatient stay by the hospital, physicians and other providers. That payment would offer at least a 3% discount to Medicare. Under this option, physicians and other providers would submit "no pay" claims to medicare and the hospital would pay them out of the single bundled payment. These arrangements may be new and maybe they are the future but they are not simple. They may not represent savings for Medicare and they certainly will complicate life for the physician. At this point it may be helpful to mention another model in health care savings that has recently become law as part of the Affordable Care Act. ACOs represent new model of health care delivery that focuses on care coordination and cost savings. This law is complicated and difficult to understand. Its object is to encompass the full continuum of care with the goal of encouraging health care providers to take collaborative responsibility for patients' overall wellbeing as opposed to just a single outcome of an intervention. Savings generated by an ACO would be shared between CMS and the ACO. with the latter distributing its portion of the savings among the participating health care providers. Under the ACO program, groups of providers can enter into a 3 year contract with CMS to share up to 10% of achieved savings over baseline Medicare spending. Participants can choose from two ACO models. Under track One, the ACO Will assume no downside risk even if it fails to achieve savings. Two allows ACOs with resources to assume some risk even if it fails and receive an increased share of the savings they accrue. In addition, specialists are not confined to participation in one ACO exclusively allowing Medicare beneficiares broader access to specialists' services. The final rule calls for all participating ACOs to comply with 33 quality measures. There are other rules about how beneficiares are assigned to private practitioners and/or a nurse practitioner. Needless to say this represents a formidable method of payment that will require study, understanding, and valuable time to digest.

GROWTH IN SPENDING

Growth in US health care spending is a topic of continual and serious discussion because of the size and persistence of the growth. We have previously alluded to the fact that the cost of medical care in this country is significantly higher than any other industrialized nation. The growth of that cost per year has become a source of great concern because much of the cost is being borne by business and the Government through its Medicare and Medicaid Programs. A short recap of what has been happening might help because some financial history is illustrative. In 2003 growth in the cost of health care was 8.1%, in 2004 it was 7.2%, in 2005 it was 6.9%. Health care spending in 2005 reached $2 Trillion or $6,697 per person. As a share of the gross domestic product health care spending increased from 15.9% in 2004 to 16% in 2005. Hospitals accounted for the largest share of overall health care costs in 2005 reaching $611.6 billion whereas spending for physician and clinical services reached $421.2 billion. Medical spending may outpace the US economy. For instance the price tag for medical assistance under Medicaid is expected to reach $674 billion over the next decade with the federal government picking up $383 billion of the cost. Medicaid program expenditures for medical assistance are expected to grow 7.9% per year for the next 10 years outpacing a 4.8% growth in the US gross domestic product. Average Medicaid enrollment is expected to increase over the next decade from 49.1 million to 55.1 million according to the Center on Budget and Policy Priorities.

Nine chronic conditions were studied to compare health care costs in a Medicaid setting. Evaluation was in 284,000 patients. Nine chronic conditions and 28 two disease combinations were evaluated. The nine chronic conditions studied were psychosis, depression, cardiovascular illness, congestive heart failure, diabetes, acid peptic illness, respiratory illness/ asthma, hypertension and anxiety. Psychosis and depression patients had the highest mean yearly costs at $6964 and $5,505respectively. Highest component costs were mental health practitioners for psychosis and hospital costs for depression. All other conditions had significantly lower yearly costs. Component costs consisted primarily of pharmacy and hospital costs. In Nov 2011 the house voted for the tax and benefits extensions and also to shield doctors from the 21% Medicare payment cut that was due to take effect June 1. The final version would still add $54.2 billion to the deficit. Medicare has been putting the squeeze on how it pays for outpatient procedures and at ambulatory surgical centers. With a 10% growth in 2007 and a 12% growth in 2006 outpatient costs are putting a squeeze on beneficiares who must make 25% co-payments. CMS proposed that that hospitals receive an average 3% increase in outpatient payments if they submit Quality data on the inpatient side. They would also report risk adjusted outcome measures including 30 day mortality for acute myocardial infarction, heart failure, and pneumonia and 3 measures from the surgical care project. Hospitals that do not submit quality data will be penalized. These are a few of the regulations that constantly stream from Medicare to control physician activity, the cost of services, and check on quality of services. While the goal is ideal the pressure on physicians and hospitals to do paper work is extreme.

TELEMEDICINE

In order to complete the number of modalities for the delivery of medical and surgical care we need to mention and elaborate on what might be the newest form of medical care to develop in the age of telecommunication and information technology to provide clinical health care at a distance. Telemedicine allows communications between patient and medical staff with both convenience and fidelity. It even allows transmission of imaging and health informatics data from one site to another. Early forms of Telemedicine have been supplemented with videotelephony and advanced diagnostic methods and additionally with telemedical devices to support in-home care. It may involve some non-clinical services involving medical education, administration and research. Telemedicine involves acquiring medical data and then transmitting this to a doctor or medical specialist at a convenient time for assessment. Dermatology, radiology and pathology are common specialties that are conducive to asynchronous telemedicine. A key difference between traditional in-person patient meetings and telemedicine encounters is the omission of an actual physical examination. The "store-and-forward" process requires the clinician to rely on a history report and audio/visual information in lieu of a physical exam. Remote monitoring enables medical professionals to monitor a patient remotely using various technical devices primarily for managing conditions such as heart disease, diabetes, or asthma. And the results are comparable to health outcomes seen in traditional in-person encounters. These encounters may also be less costly. There is an emergency telemedicine performed by SAMU Regulator Physicians in France, Spain, Chile, and Brazil. Aircraft and Maritime emergencies are also handled by SAMU centers in Paris, Lisbon, and Toulouse. Telemedicine is often used as a teaching tool since it was first introduced by MedPhone Corp in 1989. Twelve hospitals served as treatment and receiving centers in the US. Some of the more common things that telemonitoring devices keep tract of include blood pressure, heart rate, weight, blood glucose and hemoglobin as long as the patient has the right monitoring equipment. This technique should find a place for practice in remote areas and in the less developed and rural countries. There is development in the areas of telenursing and telepharmacy.

Physician Income

At some point in the exposition of medical care, manpower requirements, looming shortages, declining payments and income, and doctor burnout we need to consider physician income for the services performed. Payments, income, can vary wildly with the circumstances of the job or practice, whether it is solo, large group, clinic, hospital, medical school, foundations, charity hospitals, specialty hospitals, state government, or federal government. Jobs may be totally research, or totally managerial such as a director of a clinical service e.g. surgery for a group of hospitals or the executive director of a hospital or program. Private practice in a private office with employees involves significant overhead expenses (e.g. rent and utilities) that must be paid before "take home pay" for the practicing physician is distributed. In addition to secretary, and business manager there may be nurse, Physician Assistant, and Nurse Practitioner who usually have big salaries. And then, of course there is Malpractice Insurance which can vary up to 200,000 dollars depending on the specialty and the location of the practice. Obstetrics and Gynecology in Florida may carry the biggest price tag. One scenario was outlined by Robert DeGroote MD under the title of "The Economics of Managed Care Reimbursement" in a 2007 Bulletin of the American College of Surgeons which to this author probably represents the reality of today and the past five years. Before we consider Dr. DeGroote's experience lets look at some published physician salaries taken from computer search. While there is a long list, a look at a selected spectrum might be more helpful and interesting without losing an evaluation of the current situation. These were recorded as of 11/10/2011 and represent median salaries for some specialties.

Specialty	Median salary (USD)
Anesthesiology	331,000 to 423,000
Emergency Medicine	239,000 to 316,296

Cardiac Surgery	218,684 to 500,000
Internal Medicine	184,200 to 231,691
Obstetrics and Gynecology	251,500 to 326,924
Pediatrics	160,111 to 228,750
Family Practice	175, 000 to 220,196
Surgery (general)	284,642 to 383,333
Gastroenterology	251,026 to 396,450
Psychiatry	173,800 to 248,198
Orthopedic Surgery	397.879 to 600,000
Radiology	377,300 to 478,000
Neurological Surgery	350,000 to 705,000

It is obvious that some of the big winners are surgical specialties such as orthopedics and neurological surgery. There are illustrative charts taken from Elsevier Global Medical News that depict increases for median income of General Surgeons (47%) and for Thoracic Surgeons (22%) for the decade from 1995-2005. These amounts appear extraordinary but probably are not representative today considering the downward trend in SVUs and SGRs by the CMS (Medicare) and the reductions in reimbursement by insurance companies. It should be remembered that income is not take-home pay. The report from Robert DeGroote MD will illustrate the reality faced by doctors and in particular—surgeons dealing and working in an HMO environment. Dr. DeGroote working in a busy general and vascular surgery practice was notified that there were not enough funds in the business account to pay physician salaries. After a quick course in medical business practice and the resource-based relative value scale (RBRVS) he was able to analyze some of the problems associated with a surgical and medical practice. Doctors are usually not attuned or oriented to business practices in a profession that focuses all attention on the patient problem if you run a private practice. The surgeon does not know what are the costs and can vary widely. A business analysis in medicine or surgery relies on the principle of converting all of the payments, expenses and profits into unit values using the same relative value units (RVUs) which payers use to develop base procedural reimbursements. Each procedure has a CPT code used when submitting a bill for payment. Dividing the total collections by the total number of RVUs of service provided during that year produced left a conversion factor that was specific to that practice e.g. $36.17. The next step is to analyze costs, that is to divide the total dollar in expense by the total RVUs and arrive at CCF e.g. $29.61, this is what it cost to perform one RVU of service that year. By subtracting the CCF from the RVU one comes up with the profit for the year namely $6.59. This profit was for providing one unit of RVU to the patient. This was the global profit encompassing all payers. This was the

Medicare analysis. The same analysis was performed for the three HMOs that comprised the bulk of the managed care population, namely Aetna, United Health Care and Oxford. These three separate analysis were compared to the global analysis which was Medicare. The profit from Aetna was $4.89/RVU, Oxford was $4.76 and United was $5.63. Clearly the total profit was far less than what was received for Medicare. Using a Whipple operation as an example perhaps the single most complex operation in terms of RVUs that a general surgeon perfoms (73.72 RVUs for 2002) this translates into a profit of $485.81 for a Medicare patient, $360.49 for an Aetna patient, $350.90 for an Oxford patient, and $415.04 for a United patient. For a ruptured abdominal aneurysm (66.6 RVUs) this translates into a $439.28 profit for a Medicare patient, $325.96 for an Aetna patient, $317.30 for an Oxford patient and $ 375.29 for a United patient. For a three vessel coronary bypass graft (CABG) this translates into a $343.66 profit for Medicare, $255.01 for an Aetna patient, $248.23 for an Oxford patient, and $293.60 for a United patient. The same differences prevail for all procedures illustrating the point that none pay well or even appropriate fees for the gravity or the scope of the operation or for the effort and expertise involved. How does one stay in business in an environment that can only provide such limited income. If malpractice insurance increased $10,000 the following year he would have to perform100 extra laparoscopic cholecystectomies just to pay the increase. Increasing volume of that magnitude in a surgical practice is not a reasonable expectation. A comparison of year to year changes in Medicare reimbursements for the same operation or the same CPT#s from 1992 to 2002 shows a consistent and universal reduction in Medicare fees from 3% to 45%. the only conclusion that can be drawn from these figures is that there is a consistant reduction in fees or reimbursement for services by Medicare. The conversion factor calculated for the 50 th percentile usual and customary fee in 1993 was $86 The conversion factor for Aetna, Oxford and United is 60% less than this. The consumer price index (CPI) for medical care services (US Dept of Labor) had risen 55% from 1993 to 2003. If the conversion factor was increased the same amount the CPI for medical services would be $133.30. Comparing the conversion factors for Aetna, Oxford, and United the CPI adjusted usual and customary fee results in a decrease of 75%. Profits for the group if adjusted by the CPI were down 95%. Such changes and losses do not bode well for survival. A comparison with veterinary procedures shows that fees for similar procedures are 50-80% higher. If you compare hourly wage scales for selected specialties with those for Managed Care CEOs you find that the CEO is paid 14X more than the physicians and nurses. The message from all this math and statistics is clear if you are choosing a career path and are not independently wealthy, you better have strong altruistic desires and inclinations.

PHYSICIANS FOR A NATIONAL HEALTH PROGRAM

In 1971 Nixon proposed a health plan which would require employers to cover their workers for health care and in addition a Medicaid like program for poor families which all Americans could join by paying sliding scale premiums based on income. This plan never passed but there have been forays into providing some kind of universal health care coverage by Hillary Clinton, John Edwards and now by Barack Obama. There have been plans proposed and passed by a number of individual states such as Tennessee, Oregon and Vermont but they were either not viable or went broke under the burden of high cost. In 1988 Massachusetts became the first state to pass a version of Nixon's employer mandate, along with an individual mandate for students and the self-employed. In 1988 494,000 people in Massachusetts were uninsured. The number increased to 657,000 by2006. Oregon, in 1989 combined an employer mandate with an expansion of Medicaid and rationing of expensive care. The Governor with federal waivers promised affordable care for all but the number of uninsured remained the same. In 1992 and '93 similar bills passed in Minnesota, Tennessee, and Vermont. Minnesota's plan for universal coverage called for universal coverage by 1997 but the number of uninsured increased by 88,000. Tennessee's Democratic governor Ned McWherter found that the number of uninsured dipped for a couple years then rose higher than ever. Vermont's plan called for universal health care by 1995 but the number of uninsured has grown. The state of Washington's 1993 law included employer mandate, individual mandate for the self employed, and expanded public coverage for the poor. Over the next six years, the number of uninsured people in the state rose about 35%. As governor, Mitt Romney helped devise a health care reform. Employers that do not offer health coverage faced only paltry fines but fines on uninsured individuals escalate to $2000 in 2008. Even under the threat of fines only 7% of the 244,000 uninsured people in the state signed up. Few could afford the high premiums. Romney said "Every uninsured citizen in Massachusetts will soon have affordable health insurance ". Each of these reform efforts promised cost savings but none included real cost controls. The mandate model must include challenging insurance firms strangle on health care and recognizing that private insurance companies make universal coverage unaffordable. The inconvenient truth is that only a single-payer can save the 350 billion dollars wasted annually on medical bureaucracy and bloated executive salaries and bloated administrative costs. In 1971, New Brunswick became the last Canadian province to institute the nation's single-payer plan. Studies in the latter half of the last decade have ignited the interest in single-payer type of insurance in the US. The fallacies built into the new health care act of 2010 and some telling statistics are advancing the cause of single-payer health care for the US. The new law while it extends coverage to more people does nothing to rein in the cost which is rapidly becoming unaffordable for the country but it also does not provide universal coverage. The Physicians for a National Health Plan (PNHP) have been on the forefront, promoting, speaking, writing, agitating, contacting congressional leaders all for the sake of the present problems and what they see as the logical solution or solutions since the early 90s. There are a number of models in the in the industrialized world and we will discuss these later because many advanced industrialized societies have developed a so called single payer model of health care that is paid for and managed by the government and not by for-profit insurance companies. These are truly socialized medical care plans that work both for the patient and for the providers especially the doctors and hospitals that have lost not only income but also the freedom to practice as they see best and develop and use the new technology. If the system makes life too difficult or punishes the providers of care there will be long term consequences that will show in the numbers of doctors, nurses, and other now important providers such as nurse practitioners, and physician assistants. If the health care system is too costly for the country to support at its present level and planned universality of care, it will crumble under the weight of diminished government support or unbearable taxes.

The Canadian Health System and Thoughts on Universal Coverage

The Canadian system is the closest and perhaps the best understood system since the literature is full of analysis and because we often interact with it along the border states. Many US citizens cross over to Canada to buy their drugs because drugs are cheaper under their system. And many Canadians have crossed to the US for certain operations because there is a long waiting period in the Canadian System. Leading Canadian and US researchers confirmed that the Canadian system leads to health outcomes as good or better than the US private system at less than 50% the cost.

Canadians pay about 9% of national GDP for universal coverage compared with more than 15% of GDP to insure 85% of Americans. Kaiser Family Foundation reports that the average compound annual growth rate in US health insurance costs has been 11.6% over the past 5 years. Seventy-five percent of Americans worry about the amount they will need to pay for health insurance in the future. There is no question that restriction of supply with suboptimal access to services has contributed to the lower cost of health care in Canada. Dr. Gratzer sites waiting times in Ontario for a variety of surgery, radiation, cataract, heart, arthroplasty and imaging procedures. However there is a new approach of targeting investments to reduce waiting times. Canadians spend about 55% of what Americans spend on health care and have a longer life expectancy and a lower infant mortality. Gordan H Guyatt and colleagues did an exhaustive study on outcomes of various procedures in both Canada and the US. debating whether or not to move Canada's single-payer system towards the for-profit delivery of care. The ultimate conclusion was that the Canadian medical system is as good as the US version at least when measured by a single metric—the rate at which patients in either system died. Other people knew that Canadians live two to two and a half years longer than Americans. Overall a study by Woolhandler produced results that favored the Canadians who were 5% less likely than Americans to die in the course of treatment. Of the 38 studies the authors surveyed 14 favored Canada, 5 the US and 19 yielded mixed results. There is certainly disagreement about this and waiting times for surgery was significantly longer in Canada than the US because of a shortage of operating rooms. All these studies highlight the fact that per capita spending on health care is 89% higher in the US than in Canada. The New England Journal of Medicine in 2003 found that 31% of spending on health care in the US went for administrative costs whereas Canada spent only 17 %. The cost for health insurance for a family is now $12,000 to $14000 a year. Not many families can come up with this amount. In truth these premiums for the most part are paid by employers but premiums in some areas have risen dramatically since passage of the Affordable Care Act of 2010.(PPACA). There have been a number of suggestions and proposals that one solution for the US would be to extend Medicare coverage to all citizens instead of just those over age 65. The argument goes that the mechanism and management and economics are already worked out. On the other hand the financial problems of the country, the massive debt have promoted a reassessment of all programs especially expensive ones like Medicare and Medicaid. These two programs account for an annual budget of over a trillion dollars now which has caused fiscal hawks and budget balancers to call for dismantling Medicare and Medicaid. House republican Paul Ryan (2011) even went as far to recommend dismantling Medicare and gutting Medicaid in his zeal to save money and reduce federal expenditures. This could be labeled a cruel assault on our most vulnerable citizens. No serious assault was made on the insurance industry and their zeal to make profit and pad the bottom line. During the debates on the Affordable Health Choices Act of 2009 The Single Payer supporters were sidelined by Baucus and his colleagues most of them beneficiaries of private health industry largess. It should be noted that CEOs at the nations five largest for-profit insurance companies garnered $54.4 million in compensation in 2010. The top paid executive was Cigna's David Cordani ($15.2 million) followed by Wellpoint's Angela Braly ($13.5Million), United Healthcare's Stephen Helmsley ($10.8 Million), and Humana's Michael McCallister ($6.1 million). These represent compensation and not administrative costs which are much higher in the private insurance companies. Aministrative costs for Medicare is 4% (1.4% in 2008, excluding overhead in private Medicare Advantage and Part D pharmaceutical plans., according to the 2010 Medicare Trustees report) while administrative costs for insurance companies are above 20%.

The arguments in favor of a single payer system are many in addition to the favorable experience of the Canadian system although their system obviously needs some fine tuning.

1. In the US 60.3 million Americans (19.8%) were uninsured for at least part of 2010 up from 58.5 million in2009 according to the National Center for Health Statistics. 48.6 million Americans (16%) were uninsured at the time of the interview for the 2010 survey up from 46.3 million in2009. 35.7 million Americans (11.7%) were uninsured for more than one year. There was a slight drop in the number of uninsured children as public programs for children, primarily Medicaid and CHIP, continued to expand. Still 8.7 million children were uninsured for at least part of 2010. Nine million working-age Americans who had health insurance through a job that was lost became uninsured between 2008 and 2010 according to a survey by the Commonwealth Fund. Among those who lost employer sponsored coverage only 25% were able to find another source of coverage and only 1 in 7 were able to retain their job-based coverage through COBRA. Additionally, 32% of working age adults (49 million people) spent 10% or more of their income on health care and premiums up from 21% or 31 million adults, in 2001. In 2010, 75 million adults went without necessary health care due to cost, 73 million reported having trouble paying bills or were in medical debt, and 29 million used up all of their savings to pay medical debt. A quarter of adults with chronic conditions skipped prescriptions due to cost. (Kaiser Family Foundation).
2. Between 23 and 40 million people will remain uninsured after the federal law is fully implemented according to estimates by the Congressional Budget Office(CBO)
3. The proportion of people covered by employer sponsored private coverage fell from 69% in 2000 to 59.7 % in 2006.
15.3 million Hispanics (34.1 %) were uninsured in 2006 up 13 million from 2005
4. 90.9 million Americans (30.6%) were covered by government programs or the VA in 2006. This included 40.3 million with Medicare, (13.6%), 38.3 million with Medicaid(12.9%), 10.6 million (3.6%) with VA/Military and 1.7 million in other programs. (US Census Bureau).
5. Cancer patients face high out of pocket costs. One-third of people under 65 who are diagnosed with cancer are underinsured during or after diagnosis with 75% reporting that their lack of coverage is due to high premium costs or a pre existing condition exclusion.

6. Cancer treatment was most unaffordable for those with non-group private insurance. 43% of cancer patients with individual health insurance spent over 1/5 of their income on medical expenses. A cancer diagnosis is also a risk factor for personal bankruptcy.
7. The number of hospital emergency departments (ED) in non-rural areas declined 27% between 1990 and 2007. Safety-net hospitals, hospitals in counties with a high poverty rate and for-profit hospitals with low profitability or located in highly competitive markets are likely to close their EDs.
8. Federal revenues as a proportion of GDP are at their lowest level in 60 years. Meanwhile income inequality in the US is rising dramatically. From 1980 to 2005 more than 4/5ths of the total increase in American's incomes went to the richest 1%.
9. The economic crises has hit Hispanic and black households the hardest.
10. In the realm of costs, health care premiums will rise 8.5% in 2012 according to PriceWaterhouseCoopers survey of 1700 firms. Firms are offering employees more meager plans with higher deductibles up 13% from 2010.

COSTS FOR 2011 AND ON

US health expenditures in 2011 are projected to be $2.7 trillion, $8649 per capita, 17.7 percent of GDP. Over the next decade, health spending is predicted to grow 5.8 percent annually. In 2020 after the Patient Protection and Affordable Care Act is fully implemented health spending is projected to be 4.6 trillion, $13,709 per capita, 19.8% of GDP. (Office of the Actuary, CMS, National Health Spending Projections Through 2020)

Starbucks spent over $250 million on health insurance for its US employees, more than it spent on coffee. The total cost of health care for a family of four covered by a preferred provider plan (PPO) in 2011 is estimated to be $19,393 up 7.3% from 2010 according to Milliman Medical Index. Employer contribution accounts for 59%, $11,385, of the total while employees contribute 41% of the cost or $8,008. Employees now contribute an average of $4,728 to premiums and also pay $3,280 in out of pocket costs. (The Milliman Medical Index.)

Health spending in the US in 2006 was up 6.7% to $2.1 trillion, $7,076 per person, 16.6 per cent of GPD. The Centers for Medicare and Medicaid Services projects that in 2008 health care spending was $2.4 Trillion or $7,868 per capita and consume 16.6% of GPD (CMS, Health Affairs) Health insurance premiums grew 78% between 2002 and 2007compared with a cumulative inflation of 17%and a cumulative wage growth of 19% over the same period. The Center for Medicare and Medicaid Services (CMS) estimates that in 2017 health spending by federal and state governments will be $4.3 trillion for health coverage.(these figures exclude coverage for government employees and tax subsidies to employers)

Cherry picking is profitable to insurers because 1 percent accounts for over 20 percent of health spending. (avoiding the elderly)

CORPORATE MALFEASANCE

Health industry CEOs were richly rewarded in 2006. Without itemizing what each CEO took home for his one years effort let us say that the health industry of private insurance paid out between $5 million and $28 million dollars in annual compensation to its chief executives in the year 2006. But this was not always accompanied by stellar performance at least as far as clients (the patients) and the government are concerned. California's Health Net Inc will pay $9 million in punitive damages for cancelling the insurance policy of a woman battling breast cancer while she was in the middle of treatment. The firm claimed that she weighed more than she reported on her insurance policy, and failed to report a heart condition. The firm will also pay for misleading the state about bonuses tied to policy cancellations or 'rescission'. The firm avoided payment of $35.5 million in Medical expenses by revoking around 1600 policies between 2000 and 2006 and offering its senior cancellations analyst more than $20,000 in bonuses based on her exceeding annual targets for revoking policies. Health Net made more than $2 billion in profits in 2007.

Tampa based health insurer Wellcare is under investigation in Florida for Medicaid fraud. Almost all of the firms 4 billion in revenues comes from federal and state revenues. The firm allegedly inflated its mental healthcare costs in Florida to defraud the state of 35 million over 5years. The company is also under investigation by New York, Georgia and Connecticut officials.

Former United Health CEO William McGuire will pay $468 million to avoid charges that he manipulated stock options. McGuire resigned in2006 with stock options valued at $1.6 billion. United Health, the nations largest private insurer with 27 million enrollees faces fines up to 1.3 billion due to a failure to make timely payments on thousands of Pacificare claims in California. UnitedHealth bought Pacificare for $9.2 billion in 2006 adding three million subscribers. The California Department of Insurance uncovered 133,000 alleged violations of state laws after widespread complaints by patients and providers. Separately the State Department of Managed Care is seeking $3.5 million in fines for claims denials.

UnitedhealthGroup is under investigation by the New York Attorney General for activity at its subsidiary Ingenix, which manipulated the data that much of the insurance industry uses to determine "usual and customary" and reasonable charges. Because their limits are far below what providers actually charge patients, they are financially liable for a high proportion of any out of network care. 16 insurers have been subpoenaed in the probe that alleges that Ingenix manipulated data to artificially lower fees.

California's regulators are seeking $12.6 million in fines from Blue Shield for 1262 alleged violations of claims handling laws and regulations that resulted in more than 200 people losing their medical coverage. The state's HMO regulator is conducting a second separate investigation into the company's managed care unit with 2.3million members.

Another little known aspect of the cost and manipulation of medical care is the fact that many large corporations have health industry executives on their boards, a situation that may influence large corporations for instance from buying generic drugs instead of name brand drugs or that they may make decisions that influence legislative changes toward single payer type programs for delivering medical care.

WHERE TO FROM HERE? SOCIALIZED MEDICINE? SINGLE PAYER?

Vermont is closing in on single payer. There seems to be much discussion but little decision about how exactly the new proposed legislation is going to work. Their plan is to roll every payer they can into one system. Its easy to do with state and municipal employees but they are not sure how to do it with individual and small groups that they regulate under the terms of the Affordable Care Act. They may ask for waivers from the Obama administration so they can make use of Medicare and Medicaid money and they are trying to woo in the large national employers who are regulated by ERISA. Their plan is to tax these large employers whether they pay in or not really as a compulsion to make them join. All these payments will be run through the Vermont state government or Green Mountain Care, the single payer system. It would equalize payment rates between private insurance and Medicare and Medicaid. It would dramatically reduce paperwork and does have the support of Blue Cross and Blue Shield because it is still non-profit and never sold out to Anthem. So much for the Vermont plan. We will hear more but it is unlikely to become a model for a national single payer program.

What about support for a single payer Canadian style? A majority of physicians in the US now support legislation to establish national health insurance according to a new national survey. Similarly opposition has dropped to 32% of physicians and fewer physicians are neutral. Psychiatrists are the most supportive, followed by emergency doctors and pediatricians. In New Hampshire 67% of all physicians and 81% of all primary care physicians support single payer. A survey of small and mid sized businesses found that

60% favor a federally funded, government administered health care system financed through higher taxes. The term socialized medicine has much of its stigma but it still has a significant difference of support between democrats and republicans. Obviously democrats are more favorably inclined towards the government system.

Perhaps before we have a serious consideration of other countries and their socialized healthcare we should have a more in-depth review of

The Patient Protection and Afforable Care Act of 2010 (PPACA)

On the positive side

1. Will extend health insurance to 32 million more people by 2019
2. Provides subsidies to help many lower income Americans afford health care
3. Starting in 2014 expands Medicaid to cover 16 million more lower income people
4. Provides new funding for community health centers that could enable them to double their current capacity
5. Eliminates cost sharing for many preventive services
6. Phases out the "doughnut hole" coverage gap for the Medicare prescription drug benefit
7. Will create a new national insurance plan for long-term services: Community Living Assistance Services and Supports (CLASS) program
8. Will establish a non-profit Patient Centered Outcomes Research Institute to assess the relative outcomes, effectiveness and appropriateness of different treatments
9. Initiates some limitd reforms of the insurance industry, such as prohibiting exclusions based on pre-existing conditions and banning of annual and lifetime limits
10. Contains some provisions to improve reimbursement for primary care physicians and expand the primary care workforce

ON THE NEGATIVE SIDE OF (PPACA) THE AFFORDABLE CARE ACT

1. Surging Health care costs will not be contained as cost sharing increases for patients and their families
2. Uncontrolled costs of health care and insurance will make them unaffordable for a large and growing part of the population
3. At least 23 million Americans will still be uninsured in 2019, with tens of millions more underinsured
4. Quality of care for the US population is not likely to improve
5. Insurance "reforms" are so incomplete that the industry can easily continue to game the system
6. New layers of waste and bureaucracy, without added value, will further fragment the system
7. With its lack of price controls, the PPACA will prove to be a bonanza for corporate stakeholders in the medical industrial complex
8. Perverse incentives within a minimally regulated market-based system will lead to overtreatment with inappropriate and unnecessary care even as millions of Americans forgo necessary care because of cost
9. The reformed system is not sustainable and will require more fundamental reform sooner rather than later to rein in the excesses of the market
10. The only solution for our health care financial problems is single payer financing coupled with private delivery system. Unfortunately private practice as we now know it cannot survive the restrictions and decreasing reimbursements that the present system uses as a model. Otherwise health care will become a victim of health care for-profit corporations and an unsustainable annual increase in cost without the assurance of coverage for all citizens.

There have been discussions and proposals by a number of people that the best and perhaps the most practical solution at hand would be to put everyone on Medicare. Certainly deserves a mention and perhaps an effort to understand it as a practical solution to a very complex problem. PPACA (THE PATIENT PROTECTION AND AFFORDABLE CARE ACTOF 2010) was not designed to provide universal coverage. If it works as designed in 2019 there will still be 23 million uninsured. Employers needing financial relief will expand the trend of shifting more insurance and health care cost onto employees. Individuals buying plans in the new insurance exchanges (which won't start until2014) will discover that subsidies are inadequate to avoid financial hardship and will end up underinsured.

Medicare for all, by replacing our dysfunctional patchwork of private health insurers with a single streamlined system of financing would save about $400 billion annually in unnecessary paperwork and bureaucracy. That's enough to cover all those now uninsured and to provide every person in the United States with quality, comprehensive coverage.

Socialized Medical Care in Other Well Developed Countries

If we are to consider a more socialized system of universal health care it behooves us to look at what is being used and developed in other highly developed countries. The desire for universal health care is hardly new or unique. In the US there has been a long discussion over the years about the problems and disadvantages of what the Medical Profession has always referred to as socialized medicine inferring that if doctors worked for the government or if the government ran the system it would be 2nd rate, the doctors would be 2nd rate, and it would be the source of waste, inefficiency and reduced income. Doctors have traditionally been very independent in their private practices and resented intrusions by government or insurance companies into their decision making processes, and into their fee structure. This is not to say that the medical profession was not happy to see the era of guaranteed payments that insurance and even government brought but these advantages brought changes to the practice of medicine and the availability of medical care that are now a national social problem and loom on the national horizon as a political conundrum that must be solved. It is not only a political and social and medical problem but an escalating financial problem that threatens the stability of the national budget.

Different countries respond to the need and demand for health care in different ways but the only systems we need to examine and consider seriously are those countries that are highly industrialized and have already developed social systems that include health care. We can look to western Europe, such as England, Italy, France, and Germany, to Scandinavia such as Sweden, to Canada, to Japan, to Australia, to New Zealand and to Israel. Each has a National Health Care System that was developed in the post World War II period as they recovered. It certainly is a mixed system in the United States.

HEALTHCARE IN THE UNITED KINGDOM

In Britain it is a National System, hierarchal corporatism, with central decision making but with coverage for all. The National Health Service in England was the World's first universal health service provided by a government. It was established in 1948 by Clement Atlee' s Labor Government. Health Care in the United Kingdom is a devolved matter, meaning England, Northern Ireland, Scotland, and Wales each have their own systems of private and publicly funded healthcare. Each country having different policies and priorities has resulted in a variety of differences between the systems. Each country provides public healthcare to all UK permanent residents that is free at the point of need, being paid for from general taxation. In addition, each also has a private healthcare sector which is considerably smaller than its public equivalent, with provision of private healthcare acquired by means of private health insurance, or funded as part of an employer funded health scheme or paid directly by the customer though provision can be restricted for those with conditions such as AIDS/HIV. Taken together, the World Health Organization, in 2000, ranked the provision of health care in the United Kingdom as 15th best in Europe and 18th in the world. Overall, around 8.4% of the UKs gross domestic product (GDP) is spent on healthcare which is 0.5% below the Organization for Economic Co-operation and Development average and about one percent below the average of the European Union.

Most healthcare in England is provided by the National Health Service (NHS), England's publicly funded healthcare system, which accounts for most of the Department of Health's budget (98.6 billion pounds) in 2008-2009. The actual delivery of health care services is managed by ten Strategic Health Authorities and, below this, locally accountable trusts and other bodies. Social care services are a shared responsibility with the local NHS and the local government Directors of Social Services under the guidance of the DH. In recent years the private sector has been used to increase NHS capacity. However, since private hospitals tend to manage only routine operations and lack a level 3 critical care unit (or intensive therapy unit) unexpected emergencies may lead to the patient being transferred to an NHS hospital as very few private hospitals have a level 3 critical care unit. There are two main kinds of trusts in the NHS reflecting purchasing and provider roles such as Primary Care Trusts which examine local needs and negotiate with providers to provide health care services and provider trusts which are NHS bodies delivering health care services. Services commissioned include general practice physician services (most of whom are private businesses) working under exclusive contract to the NHS such as community nursing, local clinics, and mental health service. For most people, the majority of health care is delivered in a primary health care setting. Provider services are care deliverers, the main examples being the hospital trusts and the ambulance trusts which spend the money allocated to them by the CommissioningTrusts Hospitals, as they provide more complex and specialized care, receive the lion's share of NHS funding. Primary care is delivered by a wide range of independent contractors such as GPs, Dentists, pharmacists and optometrists which are the first point of contact for most people. Secondary care (sometimes termed acute health care) can be either elective care or emergency care and providers may be in the public or private sector, though the majority of secondary care happens in NHS owned facilities. The NHS Constitution covers the rights and obligations of patients and staff, many of which are legally enforceable. The NHS has a high level of popular support within the country and surveys show very high levels of satisfaction with the medical services received.

Each NHS system (England, Wales, North Ireland, Scotland).uses General Practitioners (GPs) to provide primary care and to make referrals to health services as necessary. Hospitals then provide more specialist care including services for psychiatric illnesses as well as direct access to Accident and Emergency Departments. Pharmacies other than those within hospitals are privately owned but have contracts with the relevant health service to supply prescription drugs. Each public healthcare system also provides free ambulance services for emergencies, when patients need the specialist transport only available from ambulance crews or when patients are not fit to travel home by public transport. These services are generally supplemented when necessary by the voluntary ambulance services. In addition patient transport services by air are provided by the Scottish Ambulance Service in Scotland and elsewhere by county or regional air ambulance trusts. In specific emergencies, air transport is also provided by naval, military, and air force aircraft. Each NHS system has its own 24-hour telephone advisory service.

In England and Wales, the National Institute for Health and Clinical Excellence(NICE) sets guidelines for Medical Practitioners as to how various conditions should be treated and whether or not a particular treatment should be funded. These guidelines are established by panels of medical experts who specialize in the area being reviewed. In Scotland, the Scottish Medicines Consortium advises the NHS Boards there about all newly Licensed medicines and formulations of existing medicines as well as the use of antimicrobiotics but doe not assess vaccines, branded generics, non-prescription-only medicines, blood products and substitutes or diagnostic drugs. Some new drugs are available for prescription more quickly than in the rest of the UK, leading to some complaints.

Cost control is the responsibility of The National Audit Office which reports annually on the summarized consolidated accounts of the NHS, and Audit Scotland performs the same function for NHS Scotland. Northern Ireland, Scotland and Wales no longer have prescription charges. However in England, a prescription charge of 7.40 pounds is payable per item, though patients under 16 years old (19 years if still in full-time education) or over 59 years are exempt from paying as are people with certain medical conditions, those on low income and those prescribed drugs for contraception. Polyclinics are being tried in England alone, in London and other suburban areas. The role of the private sector is evolving, expanding in England, and being reduced in Scotland.

Comments

The medical care system in the United Kingdom has become a model for many countries of the world. In Canada it is a Single Payer System, a Provincial system economically mandated by a national Law as universal care and in the United States we continue to have multiple forms of coverage from none to insurance, to job related health care, to government(VA, Public health), to military and military retired, to health maintenance organizations and medical management systems. We have seen hospitals merge to form corporations and enter the medical care business by providing general and specialty clinics in addition to the services provided by their emergency departments. The disarray or lack of organized clinic services to provide entry to needed care is a poignant feature of the American system for those unfortunate enough to lack insurance or to be under-insured. Some 45 million Americans fall into this category. Health Care may be divided into two segments a: health care for the individual and b: preventive medicine such as elimination of disease in a population as may have happened in the case of smallpox. Clean water and clean air, as well as safe food and vaccines become a government responsibility because of the large numbers of people involved. This aspect of health care is not under consideration when we speak of Universal Health for the individual though it is an important government function. The quality of life and the vigor of its economy and culture are directly dependent on it.

In most highly developed or well developed countries today health care is provided to everyone regardless of their ability to pay. This even extends to visitors and tourists who might find themselves with an unexpected health or accident problem. This is certainly a matter of national courtesy and service and no small matter if the country is a major tourist destination. Most countries with universal health care allow and at times even encourage private insurance and facilities.

Health Care in Italy

Another method of funding compulsory government health insurance with nominal fees is that provided by Italy which according to the World Health Organization has the second best health system in the world. England's is regarded as the best. Italy provides very low cost health care services with good standards. Doctors are well trained and private hospitals are the equal of any. There are some state hospitals in Italy that are very patchy providing comfort below what most northern Europeans and Americans expect. These hospitals are normally found in southern Italy. To avoid this, expatriates and Italians alike prefer to consider a private health insurance to generally cover the expensive costs of hospitalizations and surgeries just to have the comfort needed and to avoid waiting on long lists that are normally common in most state systems. The national health system of Italy, called the Servizio Sanitario Nazionale, provides inexpensive health care to all European citizens. This system was instituted in 1978 to provide universal healthcare for its citizens. Covered are in-patient treatments that include tests, medications, as well as surgeries and doctor visits, medical assistance that are provided by pediatricians and other specialists. The health system also provides drugs, medicines, out-patient treatments, as well as dental treatments. It is imperative to have the national health insurance called the Permesso di Soggiorno. When you register as a tourist with the local health authorities a health card and number are issued which then allows you free visits and prescriptions. If you are employed in Italy your employer is required to pay for your insurance. If you are registered with the social security system and in need of medicines or drugs your family doctor will issue you a prescription that can be presented to the pharmacy. If you have state health coverage, you qualify for those subsidized charges that reduce the cost of medicine. Otherwise, you are required to pay in full.

Hospitals in Italy. Italian state hospitals, called ospedali, can sometimes be considered as very depressing places because of poor nursing backups though some basic hospital accommodations can still be relied upon. There is a clear difference between public and private facilities though the expertise is still the same. If there is a need for you as a visitor to be hospitalized, obtain a doctors referral from your medical practitioner and there are possibilities that that your hospital charges are free. You can still have single rooms only if you pay the supplements. However there are a few hospitals that provide specialized treatments. Under the National Health you can actually request to be treated in hospitals in near cities. Italians and foreigners in Italy prefer to take private health insurance coverage over and above the basic state covers. With private insurance you can freely choose your own doctor and specialist and be treated at private hospitals. Private hospital treatments in Italy are very expensive. Other health services such as physiotherapy and counseling are available.

Health Care in Germany

In Germany health care is available to everyone. Benefits are broad and uniform and include a free choice of doctors, unlimited physician visits, free preventive checkups, no out-of-pocket payments for physician services, unlimited acute hospital care (with nominal co-payment), prescription drug coverage (with minimal co-payment), comprehensive dental benefits with minimal co-payment, vision and hearing exams, glasses, hearing aids, prostheses, inpatient psychiatric care, out-patient psychiatric care, monthly home allowances, maternity benefits, rehabilitation and occupational therapy. As of 1999 Germany immunized its children up to one year old against diphtheria, pertussis, tetanus and measles. In 1999 Germany had 287,000 active physicians including 112,683 in private practice. In 2000 the average life expectancy was 78.3 years and the infant mortality was 4 per 1000 live births. Maternal Mortality was low at 8 deaths per 100,000 live births. The German health care system has the reputation of being one of the best in the world. Medical facilities are equipped with the latest technology. They have an extensive network of hospitals and doctors that cover to the remotest areas of the country. In the WHO's year 2000 report for global healthcare Germany ranked 25th out of 191 countries based on a cost/effectiveness ratio.

The German health system is decentralized and the provision of health care in Germany is guaranteed by a large number of institutions and persons who contribute to promote, maintain and where necessary, restore the health of the population. Each of the 16 states share responsibility with the central government for the hospitals and clinics while the state regulated health insurance providers exert some control over running costs. There are numerous non-profit organizations involved in providing health care including in particular, voluntary welfare organizations such as the Arbeiterwohlfahrt (National Association for Workers Welfare), Caritas, the Deutscher Paritatischer Wohfahrtsverband (German non-Denominational Welfare Association), the German Red Cross,

Diakonisches Werk(Service Agency of the Protestant Church in Germany) etc. At the federal level, various ministries and agencies (in addition to the Federal Ministry for Health) are also responsible for health issues. In Germany there are numerous doctors that cover all specialties who work in hospitals or private practice. According to the World Health Organization (WHO) statistics Germany has an average of 358 physicians per 100,000 inhabitants. You can go straight to a specialist in Germany, however it is better to see you're your GP first as they normally have a stable of specialists they work with. All surgeons will have set hours for visiting. It is recommended that you make an appointment as waiting times can be long. But you may go without an appointment during office hours if you need urgent help. If you need major dental work you should first ask your dentist for a quote and then check it out with your insurer. Either way you should take your health insurance card with you, especially if you have to go to the hospital. Members of the statutory insurance have to pay 10 Euros per quarter to see a general practitioner since January 2004. They must contribute towards the cost of prescription drugs, wound dressings and bandages. Payments using credit cards for medical care is very rare in Germany. In general bills are sent to your home address and paid via bank account. You must keep a copy of all doctor bills for sending on to your health insurer.

HEALTH CARE IN FRANCE

The French health care system is one of universal health care largely financed by government national health insurance. In its 2000 assessment of world health care systems, the World Health Organization found that France provided the "best overall health care in the world". In 2005, France spent 11.2 % of GDP on health care, or US$3926 per capita, a figure much higher than the average spent by countries in Europe but less than the U.S. Approximately 77% of health expenditures are covered by government funded agencies.

Most general physicians are in private practice but draw their income from public insurance funds. These funds, unlike their German counterparts, have never gained self-management responsibility. Instead, the government has taken responsibility for the financial and operational management of health insurance (by setting premium levels related to income) and determining the prices of goods and services refunded. The French National Health Service generally refunds patients 70 % of most health care costs, and 100% in case of costly or long-term ailments. Supplemental coverage may be bought from private insurers, most of them non-profit, mutual insurers. Until recently coverage was restricted to those who contributed to social security (generally, workers or retirees) excluding some poor segments of the population; the government of Lionel Jospin put into place "universal health coverage" and extended the coverage to all those legally resident in France. Only about 3.7% of hospital treatment costs are reimbursed through private insurance, but a much higher share of the cost of spectacles and prostheses (21.9%), drugs(18.6%), and dental care(35.9%). (Figures from the year 2000). There are public hospitals, non-profit independent hospitals(which are linked to the public system), as well as private for-profit hospitals.

Average life expectancy in France at birth is 81 years.

The current system has undergone several changes since its foundation in 1945, though the basis of the system remains state planned and operated. Jean de Kervasdoue, a health economist, believes that French medicine is of great quality and is the only credible alternative to the Americanization of world medicine. However, despite this, Kervasdoue criticizes the fact that hospitals must comply with 43 bodies of regulations and a nit-picking bureaucracy that can be found in the system with too much regulation of the daily functions of French Hospitals. Furthermore Japan, Sweden, and the Netherlands have health care systems with comparable performance to that of France's, yet spend no more than 8% of their GDP(against France's 11.5% of GDP, or about 34 billion euros). According to various experts the battered state of the French social security system's finances is causing the growth of France's health care expenses. To control these expenses, these experts recommend a reorganization of access to health care providers, revision of pertinent laws, a repossession by CNAMTS of the continued development of medicines, and the democratization of budgetary arbitration to counter pressure from the pharmaceutical industry.

The French Health Care System: the entire population must pay compulsory health insurance. The insurers are non-profit agencies that annually participate in negotiations with the state regarding the overall funding of health care in France. There are three main funds, the largest of which covers 84% of the population and the other two a further 12%. A premium is deducted from all employees' pay automatically. The 2001 Social Security Funding Act set the rates for health insurance covering the statutory health care plan at 5.25% on earned income, capital, and winnings from gambling and at 3.95% on benefits(pensions and allowances).

After paying the doctor's or dentists fee a portion is reimbursed. This is around 75 to 85%. The balance is effectively a co-payment paid by the patient but it can also be recovered if the patient pays a regular premium to a voluntary health insurance scheme. Nationally, about half of such copayments are paid from VHI insurance and half out of pocket.

Under recent rules the general practitioners are expected to act as gate keepers who refer patients to a specialist or a hospital when necessary. However the system offers free choice of the reference doctor, which is not restricted to only general practitioner and may still be a specialist or a doctor in a public or private hospital. The goal is to limit the number of consultations for the same illness. The incentive is financial in that expenses are reimbursed at much lower rates for patients who go direct to another doctor (except for dentists, ophthalmologists, gynecologists and psychiatrists); vital emergencies are still exempt from requiring the advice from a reference doctor, who will be informed later. As costs are borne by the patient and then reimbursed, patients have freedom of choice of where to receive health care services.

Around 65% of hospital beds in France are provided by public hospitals, around 15% by private non-profit organizations, and 20% by for-profit companies.

Minister of Health and Solidarity is a cabinet position in the government of France. The healthcare portfolio oversees the public services and the health insurance part of Social Security. As ministerial departments are not fixed and depend on the Prime Minister's choice, the minister sometimes has other portfolios. In that case, they are assisted by junior Ministers.

FEES AND REIMBURSEMENTS

ACT	FEE	% REIMBURSED	PATIENT CHARGE
GENERALIST CONSULTATION	23 EURO	70%	6.6 EURO
SPECIALIST CONSULTATION	25 EURO	70%	7.50 EURO
PSYCHIATRIST CONCULTATION	37 EURO	70%	11.10 EURO
CARDIOLOGIST CONSULTATION	49 EURO	70%	14.7 EURO
ROOT CANAL	93.99 EURO	70%	28.20 EURO
PRESCRIPTION MEDICINE	VARIABLE	35-100%	VARIABLE

Medecin Generaliste: The 'medecin generaliste' (commonly called 'docteur') is responsible for patient long-term care. This implies prevention, education, care of diseases and traumas that do not require a specialist. They also follow severe diseases day-to-day (between acute crises that may require a specialist). They survey epidemics, fulfill a legal role (consultation of traumas that can bring compensation, certificates for the practice of a sport, death certificates, certificates for hospitalization without consent in case of mental incapacity) and a role in emergency care (they can be called by the SAMU, the emergency medical service) They often go to a patient's home if the patient cannot come to the consulting room(especially in case of children or old people) and they must perform night and weekend duty.

HEALTH INSURANCE (FRANCE): Because the model of finance in the French health care system is based on a social insurance model, contributions to the scheme are based on income. Prior to reform in 1998, contributions were 12.8% of gross earnings levied on the employer and 6.8% levied directly on the employee. The 1998 reforms extended the system so that the more wealthy with capital income (and not just those with income from employment) also had to contribute; since the 6.8% figure has dropped to .75% of earned income. In its place a wider levy based on total income has been introduced, gambling taxes are now redirected towards health care and recipients of social benefits also must contribute. Because the insurance is compulsory, it is effectively financed by general taxation rather than traditional insurance (as typified by auto or home insurance, where risk levels determine premiums.

The founders of the French social security system were largely inspired by the Beveridge Report in the United Kingdom and aimed to create a single system guaranteeing uniform rights for all. However, there was much opposition from certain socio-professional groups who already benefited from the previous insurance coverage that had more favorable terms. These people were allowed to keep their own system. Today, 95% of the population are covered by 3 main schemes. One for commerce and industry workers and their families, another for agricultural workers, and lastly the national insurance fund for self-employed non-agricultural workers.

All working people are required to pay a portion of their income into a health insurance fund, which mutualizes the risk of illness and which reimburses medical expenses at varying rates. Children and spouses of insured individuals are eligible for benefits, as well. Each fund is free to manage its own budget and reimburse medical expenses at the rate it saw fit.

The government has two responsibilities in this system:

- The first is a government responsibility that fixes the rate at which medical expenses should be negotiated and it does this in two ways. The Ministry of Health directly negotiates prices of medicines with the manufacturers, based on the average price of sale observed in neighboring countries. A board of doctors and experts decides if the medicine a valuable enough medical benefit to be reimbursed (note that most medicine is reimbursed, including homeopathy). In parallel, the government fixes the reimbursement rate for medical services; this means that a doctor is free to charge the fee that he wishes for a consultation or an examination, but the social security system will only reimburse it at the pre-set rate. These tariffs are set annually through negotiation with doctors' representative organizations
- The second government responsibility is oversight of health-insurance funds, to ensure that they are correctly managing the sums they receive, and to ensure oversight of the public hospital network.

Today this system is more-or-less intact. All citizens and legal foreign residents of France are covered by one of these mandatory programs, which continue to be funded by worker participation. However since 1945, a number of major changes have been introduced. Firstly, the different health-care funds (there are five: General, Independent, Agriculture, Student, Public Servants) now all reimburse at the same rate. Secondly since 2000, the government now provides health care to those who are not covered by mandatory regime (those who have never worked and who are not students, meaning the very rich and the very poor). This regime unlike the worker-financed ones, is financed via general taxation and reimburses at a higher rate than the profession based system for those who cannot afford to make up the difference.

Finally, to counter the rise in health-care costs, the government has installed two plans (in 2004 and 2006) which require most people to declare a referring doctor in order to be fully reimbursed for specialist visits, and which installed a mandatory co-payment of 1euro (about $1.45 USD) for a doctor visit, o.50 euro((about $.80 USD) for each prescribed medicine and a fee of 16-18 euro ($20-25) per day for hospital stays and for expensive procedures. Such declaration is not required for children below 16 years old (because they already benefit from another program for foreign visitors without residence in France) which will get benefits depending on existing international agreements between their own national healthcare program and the French Social Security or those benefiting from an healthcare system of French overseas territories, and for those people that benefit from the minimum medical assistance. Finally, for fees that the mandatory system does not cover, there is a large range of private complementary insurance plans available. The market for these plans is very competitive. Such insurance is often subsidized by the employer, which means that premiums are usually modest, 85% of French people benefit from complementary private health insurance. A government body, ANAES, is responsible for issuing recommendations and practice guidelines.

SPENDING: The French Healthcare system was named by the World Health Organization as the best performing system in the world in terms of availability and organization of health care providers. It is a universal health care system, but is not a single payer system. It features a mix of public and private services, relatively low expenditure, high patient success rate and low mortality rates, and high consumer satisfaction. Its aims are to combine low cost with flexibility of patient choice as well as doctors' autonomy. While 99.9 % of the French population is covered, the rising cost of the system has been a source of concern, as has the lack of emergency service in some areas. In 2004 the system underwent a number of reforms, including the "carte vitale" smart card system, improved treatment of patients with rare diseases, and efforts aimed at reducing medical fraud. While private medical care exists in

France, the 75% of doctors who are in the national program provide free care to the patient, with costs being reimbursed from government funds. Like most countries, France faces problems of rising costs of prescription medications, increasing unemployment and a large aging population.

Expenses related to the healthcare system in France represented 10.5% of the country's GDP and 15.4 % of its public expenditures. In 2004, 78.4% of these expenses were paid for by the state.

HOSPITALS: About 62%of French hospital capacity is met by publicly owned and managed hospitals. The remaining capacity is split evenly(18% each) between non-profit sector hospitals (which are linked to the public sector and which tend to be owned by foundations, religious organizations or mutual insurance associations).and by for-profit institutions.

DOCTORS: While French doctors only earn about 60% of what American doctors earn, their expenses are reduced because they pay no tuition for medical school and malpractice insurance is less costly compared to the United States.

PUBLIC PERCEPTION: Historian Paul Dutton claims that while many in the US deride the French system as "socialized" medicine, the French do not consider their mixed public and private system as "socialized" and the population tends to look down upon British and Canadian style as socialized medicine.

An Overview of the World

Other examples of universal health care that should be mentioned as established and working well are Medicare in Canada (1966)), Australia (1984) and New Zealand. Methods of payments have varied over the years but the systems have been supported by tax levies and from the general taxation. If the levy in Australia was to fully pay for the services provided, the tax would need to be set at 8% plus an additional 1% known as the Medicare Surcharge for those who do not have adequate levels of private hospital coverage. All of Europe has publically sponsored and regulated health care. Health Care in the Republic of Ireland is governed by the Health Act 2004, which established a new body to govern the National Health Service in the Republic of Ireland. The Health Institute of Slovenia was founded on March 1, 1992, after declaring independence from Yugoslavia on March 1, 1992. Most countries in Latin America provide some form of public health care provided by the government though standards and quality vary greatly and do not meet the level achieved by Europe or Canada or Australia. Cuba operates a national health system and assumes all fiscal and administrative responsibility for health care. In Asia Israel, South Korea, Seychelles, and Taiwan have Universal health care. Saudi Arabia has a publicly funded health system but the levels are low.

In Japan, payment for personal medical services is offered through a universal insurance system that provides equality of access. People without employment insurance can receive health care through programs administered through local governments. Since 1973, all elderly persons have been covered by government insurance. Patients are free to select physicians and facilities of their choice. In the early 90s there were more than a 1000 mental hospitals, 8700 general hospitals, and 1000 comprehensive hospitals with a total capacity of 1.5 million beds. In addition, 79,000 clinics offered primary out-patient services and 48,000 dental clinics were available. National health expenditures rose from about 1 trillion Yen in 1965 to nearly 20 trillion Yen in 1989 or from

5% to more than 6% of Japan's national income. Thailand, India, Sri Lanka, Philippines have plans to institute or improve government sponsored health care but as yet do not have it.

Canada has the health care system that is most closely watched and evaluated by the US in its rush to adopt or institute a universal health care system. The Federal Government of Lester B Pearson in 1966 introduced the Medical Care Act that extended the HIDS Act cost-sharing to allow each Province to establish a universal health care plan. It also set up the Medicare system. In 1984 the Canada Health Act was passed, which prohibited user fees and extra billing by doctors. In 1999, the Prime Minister reaffirmed in the Social Union Frame Work Agreement a commitment to health care that has "comprehensiveness, universality, portability, public administration and accessibility". The Canadian System is for the most part publicly funded yet most of the services are provided by private enterprises or private corporations. Most doctors do not receive an annual salary but receive a fee per visit or service. About 30% of Canadian health care is paid for through the private sector. This mostly goes for services not covered or partially covered by Medicare such as prescription drugs, dentistry and optometry. Many Canadians have private health insurance, often through employers to cover these expenses. Private services are allowed to compete by law which allows for a dual system of public and private services. In the United States a number of publically funded programs are available for those that are eligible and these programs include Medicare, Medicaid, Social Security, Veterans Health Care, Military Health, and near universal coverage mandated by some states such as Massachusetts. Tennessee instituted a form of universal health care called TennCare but could not continue it after several years because of the financial burden. This leaves a large number of citizens and non-citizens without health care coverage though many competitive Insurance companies and HMOs are available. Federal law ensures public access to emergency services regardless of ability to pay. About 45 million Americans are without insurance coverage but many more are under-insured and the trend in job related medical insurance is to reduce coverage or not offer it at all. The burden of providing fully paid medical insurance to retirees is proving to be an exorbitant burden even for mighty corporations. The cost of medical insurance and of medical care increases annually 10-15% such that purchasing an individual policy without high deductibles or with broad coverage becomes a very expensive item in the family budget.

Healthcare in Africa is almost non-existent. The out break of HIV/AIDS in Africa has crippled many populations and countries though some countries such as Uganda have been able to reduce infections unlike South Africa which denies the link between HIV and AIDS. Health care in Nigeria is a concurrent responsibility of the three tiers of government in the country. The federal government's role is mostly limited to coordinating the affairs of the university hospitals, while the state government manages the various general hospitals and local dispensaries. The total expenditure on health care as a per cent of GDP is 4.6 while the percentage of federal government expenditure is about 1.5%, a very low level. In May of 1999 the government created the National Health Insurance Scheme which encompasses government employees, the organized private sector and the informal sector. The scheme also covers children under five, permanently disabled persons and prison inmates.

Israel has a universal health care system and the Ministry of Health supervises all health matters. As of 1999 total health care expenditures averaged 9.5 % of GDP. The Arab Department of the Ministry of Health recruits public health personnel from among the Arab population and its mobile clinics extend medical aid to Bedouin Tribes in the Negev. In 2000, the infant mortality rate for the nation was 6 per 1000 live births. Life expectancy was 78 years for both men and women. The fertility rate has decreased steadily from 3.9 in 1960 to 2.8 children in 2000 for each woman during child bearing years. As of 1999 there were an estimated 3.9 physicians and 6 hospital beds per 1000 people. The Ministry of Health operates Infant Welfare Clinics, nursing schools, and laboratories. The largest medical organization in the country, the Workers Sick Fund administers hospitals, clinics, convalescent homes and mother-and-child welfare stations. Immunizations for children up to one year old were: diphtheria, pertussis, tetanus, polio and measles. Aids was low and tobacco consumption down.

Switzerland is a nation that has successfully attained universal coverage by mandating that individuals buy private insurance. Yet Switzerland's mandate program resulted in only minute increases from before the mandate when 98-100% of the population had coverage. Private health insurers in Switzerland are non-profit unlike their American counterpart. They are non-profit and do not set premiums benefits or fees to providers and operate as quasi-government agencies. The Dutch on the other hand estimate that their reform that allowed their non-profit regional sickness funds to convert to a for-profit status and new insurers to begin marketing private coverage in the Netherlands has left hundreds of thousands without coverage. About 241,000 are not enrolled in a health plan and another 240,000 have already defaulted on their premiums including a higher proportion of seniors, the unemployed and single parent families out of a population of 16.4 million.

USA experiments with state systems. TennCare was the state of Tennessee's health care insurance plan designed to expand health insurance through the state's Medicaid program by utilizing managed care. Launched in 1994 it was hoped that it would solve access to affordable health care insurance and a Medicaid budget that was fast consuming the largest portion of the state budget. It was supposed to be budget neutral and require no greater federal funding than the previous Medicaid program. The state sought to achieve this by replacing Medicaid-fee-for service payment method with a managed care model. In its first year of operation it quickly grew to the federal cap of 1.5 million people. In response to this growth the state closed eligibility to adults who were uninsured. In its first five years TennCare saved the state money. But then problems began to develop related to the operation of the seven managed-care organizations (MCOs) and physicians complained that they were not being paid. The state was forced to take over the failing managed care organizations and health care providers were left with millions in unpaid bills. By 1999 it was clear that reform was need. State Officials tried to route more money to the providers in the form of monthly capitation payments but the MCOs were unable to make it. In2002 the state's waiver agreement with the federal government was renewed though CMS would not agree to many of the original funding mechanisms making the program even less cost-effective. By 2002 it became clear that the program as structured was not viable and threatened the fiscal health of the state. The governor moved to return to the traditional Medicaid while preserving coverage for all children. By 2005 approximately 160,000 people who were not Medicaid eligible were removed from TennCare. At that time Tennessee was one of half dozen states in the nation with no limits on pharmacy benefits. The state set limits at five prescriptions with exclusions for children, pregnant women, nursing homes, and emergency care. Limits were also placed on doctors' visits and hospital stays. This illustrates some of the dangers and results of state plans.

The Massachusetts Health Care Reform was enacted in 2006 and requires nearly every resident of Massachusetts to obtain or purchase health insurance coverage. This is an example of a trend in health care coverage that is becoming common in some states as a method of tackling health care on a universal basis. It requires nearly every resident to obtain or purchase health insurance coverage or pay a penalty. The law provides free health care for residents earning less than the federal poverty line and subsidized access for those earning up to three times the poverty threshold. The incentives to comply include a new quasi public regulatory authority, 'The Commonwealth Health Insurance Connector Authority' which may impose penalties for failing to comply such as loss of the $219 individual Massachusetts annual income tax exemption. As of March 2006 there were around 497,900 uninsured residents of Massachusetts. These low income and underinsured residents commonly use the emergency room as a source of medical care because of their lack of insurance.

Similar activities have been taking place in Pennsylvania where Governor Rendell called on lawmakers to use part of their medical malpractice fund as part of legislation to extend insurance subsidies for 2008. Extending the health care initiative to roughly 800,000 uninsured adult Pennsylvanians has been stalled by opposition to a payroll tax. The health insurance would also be financed by Medicaid dollars and premiums that would be paid by small businesses. California, Maine and Vermont are also attempting to implement universal health systems at the state level. San Francisco is attempting this at a city wide level.

This leads us to the all important consideration of cost. The methods used to cover the cost of universal health care are as varied as the number of countries that have had the courage to undertake it politically. Taxation is the basic method used but the source of the taxes are as varied as the organizational realities of the government. The realities of funding health care in the United States is the high cost as part of the GDP. Insurance companies and managed care enterprises do attempt to sell to low risk clients. This limits the ability of patients with chronic diseases and permanent disabilities to obtain much needed care. On the other hand the rise in cost and the portion of the GDP that now goes into health care to say nothing of the expected 12% increase expected this year cannot but force a vigorous debate not on the merits of universal care but of the necessity for controlling costs. A comparison of life statistics, per capita costs, and percent of GDP that is devoted to health care, clearly reveals that the USA has the lowest life expectancy of the industrialized nations, the highest per capita cost ($5711 vs $2801), the highest portion of its GDP devoted to medical care (15.2% vs 9.4%), and the highest portion of government revenue spent on health (18.5% vs 16.05%). Finally the per cent of health care costs paid for by the government shows most countries pay between 67.5 % (Australia) and 85.7% (UK) whereas the US pays 44.6%.

In the United States certain publically funded health care programs help to provide for the elderly, disabled, military service families, veterans, children and the poor. Federal Law ensures public access to emergency services. However a system of universal health care has not been implemented and some 44 million Americans are without health insurance coverage. Bills resulting from medical care is a common cause if not the most common cause of family bankruptcies. The politics and the financial mechanisms of providing universal coverage are so complex at the present time that there is little chance there will be agreement on plan, taxes, legislative agenda, and the myriad of details such as organization, role of physicians, role of private practice, managed care plans, and all the ancillary services that are needed such as dental care, optometry and glasses, immunizations, assisted living, prostheses, chairs and mobility, special beds, home care, nursing care and mental health, along with the facilities, clinics, hospitals, pharmacies, and highly specialized units for advanced techniques and equipment.

In conclusion many industrialized countries have developed systems of health care to which all the people have equal access. There are critics of some plans such as delays in getting certain procedures or operations done but there is no indication that the people want to give up or change their system except to improve it. The election of Barach Obama as President of the United States along with a preponderance of democrats in congress and the campaign emphasis on solving the medical care problems in the US has resulted in passage of a law that portends serious legislative proposals in the direction of a more socialistic method of providing medical care for all.

1. The commonwealth fund conducted its thirteenth annual health policy survey (2010) and the findings found that US adults were the most likely to incur high medical expenses spend more time on paperwork and have more claims denied. Before we revue some of the major industrialized countries it might be helpful to review some differences by Chris Fleming. The countries surveyed were Australia, Canada, France, Germany, the Netherlands, New Zealand, Norway, Sweden, Switzerland, The United Kingdom, and the United States.
2. Twenty per cent of US adults said they had had serious problems paying medical bills in the previous year. Responses to the same question from the other ten countries were in the single digits. US respondents were also more likely than adults in other countries to have gone without care because of cost
3. Thirty-five percent of US adults had out of pocket medical spending of $1000 during the previous year, a far higher percentage than any other country.
4. A lower proportion of adults in the United States (70%) than in all the other countries except Sweden (67%) and Norway (70%) were confident that they would receive the most effective treatment when needed.
5. When asked about access to prompt medical care, 57% of US adults said they had seen a doctor or nurse the same or the next day the last time they were sick and needed care. Switzerland had the most rapid access(93%) Adults in three other countries (Canada, Norway, and Sweden) reported longer waits than the US adults.
6. Nearly one third of US adults (31%) reported either denial of payments by insurers or time consuming interactions with insurers, a higher rate than in all other countries. Twenty-five percent of US respondents reported that their insurance company denied payment or did not pay as much as expected; 17% said that they spent a lot of time on

paperwork or disputes for medical bills or insurance—the highest rates in the survey.
7. The United States had the widest and most pervasive differences in access and affordability by income of the eleven countries. The United Kingdom had the least.

A review of other large and well developed countries should help to frame the debate since the US is about to embark on a whole new medical care plan that combines private insurance, government sponsored insurance for the elderly and very poor (CMS), plus but importantly The VA Health care system, the Military System, TRICARE for retired military and the Public Health Hospitals that provide Indian and sea-faring services. This offers a lot but combined it represents the most expensive system with results that don't compare well with some of the other systems we will look at.

HEALTH SYSTEMS IN SOME FOREIGN COUNTRIES

THE HEALTH IN BELGIUM

The health care system in Belgium is funded through the state sickness fund. There are four tiers of operation consisting of central government, national associations, federations of local societies, and local mutual aid societies. The Belgian government believes that this power sharing motivates each local fund to work hard to attract and satisfy its members. In Belgium health insurance is mandatory. Basic is provided by the national social security system which is known as the mutualite or ziekenfonds. Contributions are paid by both employers and employees and they amount to 7.35% of each person's gross salary. The employee must pay 3.55 % directly from their wages and employers must pay the other 3.8%. Self employed must pay the whole 7.35% on a quarterly basis. Cover is automatically provided for unemployed dependent family members and children up to the age of 18. The unemployed, old age pensioners, and people on long-term sickness benefit or maternity leave do not have to pay healthcare contributions. Foreigners immigrating to Belgium without jobs must produce proof of private health insurance in order to obtain their residence permit. For historic reasons some funds are limited to members of various religious, political or professional groups, but most funds are open to everyone. Each fund charges the same basic contributions well as providing similar benefits, but some take longer to repay the fees. People have to wait 6months before they are able to claim benefits unless they previously belonged to a health scheme as a dependent or if they were covered by a state health care plan in another EU country for at least six months before their arrival in Belgium. People have to pay a certain amount of their medical bill themselves and they usually pay fees directly to their doctor or the hospital. They must submit their receipts for reimbursement and the money is paid directly into their bank account. Most Belgians take out supplementary health insurance for the portion of the bill that is not covered as an employment benefit.

HEALTHCARE IN NORWAY

Norway has an excellent standard of compulsory state funded healthcare. Medical staff are extremely well trained and healthcare is available to all citizens and registered long-term residents. Private healthcare is also available. The ministry of health determines healthcare policy and oversees the state system. Healthcare policy is executed by five health regions and the municipalities. The health service in Norway is funded predominantly through taxes taken directly from salaries and there is no specific health contribution fund. The National Insurance Administration known as the Trygdeetaten is responsible for the national insurance scheme NIS, a state insurance scheme that guarantees everybody a basic level of welfare. The NIS provides benefits for illness, accidents, bodily defects, pregnancy, birth, disability, death, and loss of the breadwinner as well as for unemployment and old age. All citizens who live or work in Norway or are on permanent work within the Norwegian continental shelf must contribute to the NIS. In addition people living in Svalbard (Spitzbergen) and Jan Mayen who are employed by a Norwegian employer or were insured under the National Insurance act prior to their stay in these areas and certain categories of Norwegian citizens working abroad must pay compulsory National Insurance contributions. Employees and the self-employed become members of the social security system through payment of National Insurance. Those who do not fulfill these requirements can apply for voluntary membership in the NIS if their stay exceeds 3 months. Students from Scandinavian countries and Iceland become members of the Norwegian NIS if they register as residents of Norway. Students from other countries automatically qualify for healthcare if they study in the country for over a year.

HEALTH CARE IN SWEDEN

Everyone in Sweden has equal access to health-care services. The Swedish health-care system is taxpayer funded and largely decentralized. The system performs well in comparison with other countries and life expectancy continues to rise (79 years for men and 83 years for women).

In the Swedish Health-Care system, responsibility for health and medical care is shared by the central government, city councils and municipalities. The Health and Medical Service Act regulates the responsibilities of the county councils and municipalities. Responsibility for providing health care is decentralized to the county councils and in some cases to the municipal government. County councils are political bodies whose representatives are elected by their residents every four years on the same day as national general elections. County councils are also responsible for dental care for local residents up to the age of 20. Sweden's municipalities are responsible for care for the elderly in the home or in special accommodation. Their remit includes care for people with physical disabilities or psychological disorders. Municipalities are also responsible for providing support and services for people released from hospital care as well as school health care. Sweden is in the midst of a national effort to ensure that patients are protected from accidents, incorrect treatments, and other incidents. Another goal is to halve the incidence of health care related infection by 2010

Waiting times for preplanned care, such as cataract, or hip-replacement surgery have long been a cause of dissatisfaction. As a result, Sweden has introduced a health-care guarantee namely that no patient should have to wait more than 90 days once it has been determined what care is needed. If the time limit expires the patient is offered care elsewhere; additional costs are paid for by their own county council. The situation has improved and the central government has allocated an extra billion Kroner for the services. Costs for health and medical care are about 9 per cent of Sweden's gross domestic product (GDP) and this has remained stable since the 1980s. The bulk of health and medical costs are paid for by county councils and municipal taxes. Contributions from the national government are another source while patient fees cover only a small percentage of costs. County council costs in 2008, excluding dental care, were up 5.2% and primary care accounts for the largest increase in costs. It has become more common for county councils to buy services from private health care providers (about 10%) under the same regulations and fees that apply to municipal care facilities.

Most care in Sweden today is provided in health centers where a variety of health professionals: doctors, nurses, midwives, physiotherapists, and other staff work. Patients are able to choose their own doctors. There are special clinics for children and expecting mothers as well as youth clinics, and family planning clinics. In 2009 they introduced a primary choice system in primary care that allows patients choosing whether they would prefer to go to a private or public health center. All health care providers that meet requirements are entitled to start a health center that is reimbursed with public funds. Sweden has 60 hospitals that provide specialist care with emergency services 24 hours a day. Eight of these are regional hospitals where highly specialized care is offered and where most teaching and research is based.

HEALTH CARE IN POLAND

Poland's health care system is based on general health insurance. Persons covered by the general health insurance are entitled to free health services in the territory of Poland. Rules of the general health insurance are provided in the law of 23 January 2003 on the General Insurance in the National Health Fund. An insured person and members of his family are entitled to free health care in case they receive these services at health care providers who have concluded contracts on providing health services with the regional branch of the National Health Fund (NFZ) The contract for providing health services specifies the kind and the scope of the services contracted by the given health provider with the National Health Fund. Health care providers who have a contract for providing health services can be identified by a board with NFZ logo situated outside the building. The regional branch office of the NFZ has information on all physicians who belong to the NFZ. The National Health Fund is responsible for assuring health services for injured persons and members of their family. The Fund finances health services and assures refunds for medicines. Health care providers are: doctors, dentists, hospitals, first aid stations dispensaries, health centers, out-patient clinics, and both individual and group specialists. Emergency Medical Services is a service of public pre-hospital health care including ambulance service provided by individual Polish cities and counties. These services are provided by the local publicly operated hospital and funded by the government of Poland, however there are private-for profit ambulance services. In case of necessity a visitor from a member European country temporarily is entitled to free care on the basis of form E 111 issued in his country or the European Health Insurance Card otherwise the patient is obliged to cover the cost himself. In case of need of a specialist treatment a referral by the doctor who practices within the health care system is needed. The majority of the costs of dental services is the responsibility of the patient. However a patient who presents form E111, the European Health Insurance card or a certificate receives free dental services.

HEALTHCARE IN RUSSIA

Russia has more physicians, hospitals, and health care workers than almost any other country in the world on a per capita basis. However since the collapse of the Soviet Union, the health of the Russian population has declined considerably as a result of social, economic, and life style changes. As of 2009 the average life expectancy in Russia was 62.7 years for males an 74.6 for females. The average life expectancy of 68.6 years at birth is nearly 10 years shorter than the overall average figure for the European Union. There is a gender imbalance with more women than men, an imbalance that is the result of World War II, where Russia lost more men than any other nation in the world. In 2008, 57% of all deaths were caused by cardiovascular disease. The second leading cause of death was cancer. External causes of death such as suicide, road accidents, murders, alcohol poisoning, and others claimed 244,463 lives (11%). Other causes of death ran the usual mixture of digestive, respiratory, infectious diseases, and tuberculosis (1.2%). The infant mortality rate was 8.5 deaths per 1000 down from 9.6 in 2007. There has been a dramatic rise of both cases and deaths from Tuberculosis.

There are major problems that arise from life styles. These include smoking, alcohol consumption, HIV/AIDS, and suicide. Russia is the world leader in smoking according to survey published in 2010 by Russia's Health and Social Development Ministry. 43.9 million adults in Russia are smokers. Among Russians aged 19 to 44 years 7 in 10 smoke and 4 in 10 women smoke. It is estimated that 330,000-400,000 die in Russia each year due to smoking related diseases. Alcohol consumption and alcoholism are major problems in Russia. HIV/AIDS have become major problems due to the explosive growth of intravenous drug use. At the end of 2007 there were 416,113 registered cases but the actual number is estimated at 940,000. The Russian Federation has demonstrated a high level of commitment in response to the AIDS epidemic.

Russia also has one of the highest suicide rates in the world although it has been steadily decreasing.

Pre-1990s Soviet Russia had a totally socialist model of health care. The new Russia(1991-1993) has changed to a mixed model of health care with private financing and provision running alongside state financing and provision. Article 41 of the 1993 constitution confirmed a citizen's right to healthcare and medical assistance free of charge. This is achieved through compulsory medical insurance rather than just tax funding. This and the introduction of new free market providers was intended to promote efficiency and patient care. The OECD reported that unfortunately none of this has worked as planned and in some ways it has made the system worse. The populations health has deteriorated on virtually every measure. The resulting system is overly complex and very complex. Private structures have proven to be woefully inadequate. Although there are more than 300 private insurers and numerous public ones in the market real competition for patients is rare leaving most patients with little or no effective choice of insurer, and in many places no choice of health care provider either. The insurance companies have failed to develop as active, informed purchasers of health care services. Most are passive intermediaries, making money by simply channeling funds from regional OMS funds to healthcare providers. After Vladimir Putin became president in 2000 there was a significant growth in spending for public healthcare; life expectancy increased and infant mortality decreased. Russian Prime Minister Putin announced a large scale health-care reform in 2011 and pledged to allocate more than $300 billion rubles ($10 billion) to improve health care in the country. He also raised the obligatory medical insurance tax paid by companies. There has also been an effort to increase the birth rate because of Russia's demographic crises. In 2007 Russia saw the highest birth rate since the collapse of the USSR. Immigration is also viewed as necessary to sustain the country's population.

HEALTH CARE IN TURKEY

Health Care in Turkey used to be dominated by a centralized state system run by the Ministry of health. In 2003 the governing Justice and Development Party introduced a sweeping health reform program aimed at increasing the ratio of private to state health provision and making health care available to a larger share of the population. Private care has blossomed in Turkey in the last decade due to the long queues and poor personal service in state run hospitals. Most private hospitals have contracts with various insurance companies so it is now possible to get better treatment. After rising competition from the private hospitals there has been an increase in the quality of state hospitals. At 7.6% of GDP in 2005 Turkey's public expenditure on national health was below that of other developed countries. In the early 2000s about 63% of expenditures came from public sources. In 2006 there was one doctor for every 700 people one nurse for every 580 people and one hospital bed for every380 people. The rural population is poorly served by the health-care system which is much more developed in the western half of the country. Between 80-90% of the population including self-employed workers have health care provided by the national pension system, but the low quality of care encourages the use of private health providers in urban areas. Only about 2% of the population, mainly in the urban areas, has private health insurance. In 2005 about 75% of private health expenditures were out of pocket rather than covered by health insurance. The most frequent causes of death are infectious and parasitic diseases but the incidence of many of these has decreased sharply because of the improved availability of potable water. The availability of inoculations for children has increased and the infant mortality rate is down sharply. HIV remains a problem for a small segment of the population.

Public Health-Care in China

China is undertaking reform of its health-care system. The New Rural Co-operative Medical Care System (NRCMCS) is a 2005 initiative to overhaul the healthcare system, particularly intended to make it more affordable for the rural poor. Under the NRCMCS, the annual cost of medical coverage is 50 yuan (US $7) per person. Of that, 20 yuan is paid by the central government, 20 yuan by the provincial government, and a contribution of 10 yuan is made by the patient. As of September 2007, around 80% of the rural population of China had signed up (about 685 million people) The system is tiered depending on the location. If patients go to a small hospital or clinic in their local town the system will cover roughly 70-80-% of their bill. If the patient visits their county clinic, the percentage of the cost being covered falls to about 60%. If the patient requires a specialist in a modern city hospital the plan would cover about 30% of the bill.

Indicators of the status of China's health sector can be found in the nation's fertility rate of 1.8 children per women and an infant mortality rate of 25.3 per 1000 live births. In 2005 China had about 1,938,000 physicians (1.5per 1000 persons) and about 3, 074,000 hospital beds.(2.4 per 1000 persons). Health expenditures were US $224 per capita, or 5.5% of GDP. Some 37% of public expenditures were devoted to health care in China in 2001 However, about 80% of health and medical care services are concentrated in cities and timely care is not available to more than 100 million people in rural areas. To offset this China has a 5year plan to invest 20 million renminbi ($2.4 billion) to rebuild the rural medical service.

China has a long history of traditional medicine, probably the longest of any existing civilization. The methods and theories have developed for over 2000 years. Western medical theory and practice came to China in the nineteenth and twentieth century notably through the efforts of missionaries and the Rockefeller Foundation, which together founded the Peking Union Medical

College. Today Chinese Traditional Medicine is practiced alongside western medicine. And physicians who have received training in western medicine will provide both types of medicine as primary care givers in the rural clinics of China. Western Medicine has gained increasing acceptance particularly in the 1970s and 1980s when the number of physicians and physician assistants increased by 225,000. In 1981 there were reportedly 516,000 senior physicians trained in western medicine and 290,000 senior physicians trained in traditional Chinese medicine. In general there is some combining of both but the two are generally practiced in separate departments. Traditional medicine depends on herbal treatments, acupuncture, acupressure, burning of herbs over acupuncture points, Cupping (local suction of skin), qigong (coordinated movements, breathing, and awareness, (Tui Na (massage), and other culturally unique practices.

After 1949 the Ministry of Public Health was responsible for all health care activities and established and supervised all facets of health policy. Along with a system of national, provincial, and local facilities the ministry regulated a network of industrial and state enterprise hospitals and other facilities covering the health needs of workers in these enterprises. In1981 this additional network provided approximately 25% of the country's total health services. The post 1990 history of medical care in China is based on the development of western style medical facilities with international staff with up-to-date medical technology and physicians who are both knowledgeable and skilled. Most VIP wards also provide medical services to foreigners and have English speaking doctors and nurses. Emerging public health problems are the result of pollution, progressing HIV problem, and hundreds of millions of cigarette smokers, and an increase of obesity. Hepatitis B is endemic. Avian flu outbreaks are an ever present danger. Pig human transmission of streptococcus suis bacteria led to 38 deaths in Sichuan. As of 2004 in more undeveloped areas it is advisable to drink only bottled water because of cholera dangers. Tuberculosis is a major health problem in China which has the second largest tuberculosis epidemic after India. Many social ills still remain, one of them is malnutrition amongst rural children. Water supply and sanitation facilities are still a problem in parts of China. Equitable health care across the spectrum for the population at large is still a problem. China's first case of the highly contagious disease SARS, (severe acute respiratory syndrome) occurred in Guangdong in 2002 and within 3 months the ministry of health reported 300 cases and 5 deaths in the province.

HEALTH CARE IN NEW ZEALAND

1. The health care system in New Zealand has undergone significant changes throughout the past several decades. From an essentially fully public system in the early 20th century, reforms have introduced market and health insurance elements primarily in the last three decades, creating a mixed public-private system for delivering healthcare.
2. The Accident Compensation Corporation covers the cost of treatment for cases deemed 'accidents', including medical misadventure, for all people legally in New Zealand (including tourists) with the costs recovered by levies on employers, employees and some other sources such as car registration.
3. The relatively extensive and high quality system of public hospitals treats citizens or permanent residents free of charge and is managed by district health boards. However, costly or difficult operations often require long waiting list delays unless the treatment is medically urgent. Because of this, there is a secondary market of health insurance schemes which fund operations and treatment for their members privately. Southern Cross Health Insurance, a non-profit-scheme is the largest of these at about 60% of the health insurance market and covering almost a quarter of all New Zealanders in 2007, even operating its own chain of hospitals.
4. Primary-care (non-specialist doctors/family doctors) and medications on the list of the New Zealand government agency PHARMAC require co-payments, but are subsidized, especially for patients with community health *service cards or higher user health cards.*

Emergency services are primarily provided by St. John New Zealand charity (as well as Wellington Free Ambulance in the Wellington Region), supported with a mix of private (donated) and public (subsidy) funds.

In 2005, new Zealand spent 8.9% of GPD on health care or US$2,403 per capita. Of that approximately 77% was government expenditure. In a 2010 study New Zealand came in last in a study for the level of medications use in 14 developed countries (i.e. used least medicines overall) and also spent the least amount on healthcare amongst the same list of countries, with US$2510 per capita(new Zealand), compared to the United States at US$7290.

The Ministry of Health is responsible for the oversight and funding of the twenty District Health Boards (DHBs). These are responsible for organizing health care in the district and meeting the standards set by the Ministry of Health. Twenty-one DHBs came into being on Jan 1, 2001 with Southland and Otago DHBs merging into Southern DHB on1 May 2010. The boards for each DHB are elected in elections held every 3 years, with the exception of one of the eight board members, who is appointed by the ministry of health.

The DHBs oversee the forty-six Primary Health Organizations established throughout the country. These were set up in July, 2002., with a mandate to focus on the health communities. Originally there were 81 of these but this has been reduced down to 46 in 2008. They are funded by DHBs, and are required to be entirely non-profit, democratic bodies that are responsive to their communities needs. Almost all New Zealanders are enrolled in a PHO, as there are financial incentives for the patients to become enrolled.

Public vs private payment. The burden for the core of the health care system rests with government expenditure (approx 77%), Private payment by individuals also plays an important role in the overall system although the cost of these payments are comparatively minor.

Damage a result of accidents, ranging from minor to major physical and psychological trauma is generally completely covered by the Accident Compensation Corporation (ACC) This may include coverage for doctors visits and lump-sum payments. Those earning less than certain amounts, depending on the number of dependents in their household can qualify for a Community Services Card. (CSC), which reduces the upfront fee for visiting a doctor. Hospital and specialist care, on the other hand, is totally covered by the government if the patient is referred by a general or family practitioner.

Some health care statistics for New Zealand: life expectancy for females-82, life expectancy for males-78, neonatal mortality per 1000 live births-3, abortion is legal in New Zealand, there are approximately 2000 drugs listed on the national schedule that are either fully or partially subsidized.

HEALTH CARE IN AUSTRALIA

Health care in Australia is provided by both private and government institutions. The Minister for Health and Ageing administers national health policy, elements of which, such as hospitals are overseen by individual states. In Australia the current system, known as Medicare, was instituted in 1984. It coexists with a private health system. Medicare is funded partly by a 1.5% income tax levy but mostly out of general revenue. An additional levy of 1% is imposed on high income earners. An additional 1% levy is imposed on high income earners without private health insurance. In addition to Medicare there is a separate Pharmaceutical Scheme that heavily subsidizes prescription medication. In2007-8, Australia spent 9.1%of GDP on health care, or $4874 per capita.

Health care in Australia is universal. The federal government pays a large percentage of the cost of services in public hospitals. The government subsidizes Medicare services typically:100%of in-hospital costs; 75%of general practitioner cost and 85% of specialist services. Where the government pays the large subsidy, the patient pays the remainder out of pocket, unless the provider of the service chooses to use bulk billing, charging only the scheduled leaving the patient with no extra costs. In some countries this commonly referred to as copayment. Where a particular service is not covered, such as dentistry, optometry and ambulance transport the patient must pay the full amount. (unless they hold a Low Income Earner Card, which may entitle them to subsidized access.) Individuals can take out private health insurance to cover out-of-pocket costs with either a plan that covers just selected services, to a full coverage plan. In practice a person with private insurance may still be left with out-of-pocket payments as services in private hospitals often cost more than the insurance payment. The government encourages individuals with income above a set level to privately insure. This is done by requiring those individuals to pay a surcharge of 1% of income if they do not take out private insurance

The public health system in Australia is called Medicare which funds free universal access to hospital treatment.

. It is funded by a 1.5% tax levy on taxpayers with incomes above a threshold amount, an extra 1% levy on high income earners without private health insurance. The private health insurance system is funded by a number of private health insurance organizations. The largest of which is Medibank Private, which is government owned but operates as a government business enterprise under the same regulatory regime as all other registered private health funds. Some private health insurers are "for-profit" enterprises and some are non-profit organizations such as HCF Health Insurance. Some have membership limited to particular groups. Some focus on specific regions—like HBF which centers on western Australia, but the majority have open memberships set out in the PHIAC annual report. Most aspects of private health insurance in Australia are regulated by the Private Health Insurance Act, 2007. Complaints and reporting of the private health industry is carried out by an independent government agency, the private Health Insurance Ombudsman. The private health system in Australia operates on a "community rating" basis whereby premiums do not vary solely because of a persons previous medical history, current state of health or their age. Balancing this are waiting periods in particular for pre-existing conditions. Funds are entitled to impose a waiting period of up to 12 months on benefits for any medical condition the signs and symptoms of which existed during the six months ending on the day the person first took out insurance. This also includes obstetrical conditions.

The Australian government has introduced a number of incentives to encourage adults to take out private hospital insurance:

1. Lifetime Health Cover. If they have not taken out private hospital insurance by their 31st birthday their premiums will include a loading of 2% per annum
2. Medicare levy surcharge: People whose taxable income is greater than a specified amount (currently $70,000 for singles and $140,000 for couples) and who do not have an adequate level of private hospital cover must pay a 1% surcharge on top of the standard 1.5% Medicare Levy
3. Private Health Insurance Rebate: The government subsidizes the premiums for all private health insurance cover, including hospital and ancillary (extras), by 30%, 35% or 40%. The Labor Government under Kevin Rudd announced that as of June 2010, the rebate would become means-tested and offered on a sliding scale.

PROGRAMS Medicare Australia is responsible for administering Medicare (Australia), which provides subsidies for health services. It is primarily concerned with the payment of doctors and nursing staff, and the financing of state-run hospitals. The Pharmaceutical Benefits Scheme provides subsidized medications to patients. Low-income earners may receive a card that entitles the holder to cheaper medicines under the PBS. There are: A National Immunization Program Schedule that provides many immunizations free of charge by the federal government; the Australian Organ Donor Register, a national register which registers those who elect to be organ donors. Registration is voluntary in Australia and is commonly recorded on a drivers license or proof of age card are also managed by the federal government.

The Therapeutic Goods Administration is the regulatory body for medicines and medical devices in Australia. At the borders the Australian Quarantine and Inspection station is responsible for maintaining a favorable health status by minimizing risk from goods and people entering the country. The Australian Institute of Health and Welfare is Australia's national agency for health and welfare statistics and information. The Institute publishes over 140 reports each year on various aspects of Australia's health and welfare.

Each state is responsible for the operation of public hospitals.

The Australian Red Cross collects blood donations and provides them to Australian healthcare providers. Other health services such as medical imaging (MRI etc) are often provided by private corporations but patients can still claim from the government if they are covered by the Medicare Benefits Schedule.

Quality of Care: In an international comparative study of health care systems in five countries (Australia, Canada, Germany, New Zealand, and the United States) found that Australia ranks highest on healthy lives, scoring first or second on all the indicators, although its overall ranking in the study was below the UK and Germany systems, tied with New Zealand's and above those of Canada and the US. A global study of end-of-life care conducted by the Economist magazine, published the compared end-of-life care, gave the highest ratings to Australia and the UK out of the 40 countries studied, the two country's systems receiving a rating of 7.9 out of 10 in an analysis of access to services, quality of care, and public awareness.

Aboriginal Australians are much less healthy than the rest of the Australian community

Cigarette smoking is the largest preventable cause of death and disease in Australia. Australia has one of the highest proportions of overweight citizens in the developed nations in the world.

HEALTH CARE IN INDONESIA

Indonesia has a very primitive system of health care. Unsafe drinking water is a major cause of diarrhea which is a major killer of young children in Indonesia.

Indonesia had a three tiered system of community health centers in the late 1990s, with 0.66 hospital beds per 1000 population, the lowest rate among members of the Association of Southeast Asian Nations (ASEAN). In the mid-1990s, according to the World Health Organization there were 16 physicians per 100,000 population in Indonesia, 50 nurses per 100,000 and 26 midwives per 100,000. Both traditional and modern practices are employed. Government health expenditures are about 3.7% of the gross domestic product (GDP). There are about a 75:25 per cent ratio of public to private health-care expenditures.

HIV/AIDS has posed a major public health threat since the early 1990s. In2003 Indonesia ranked third among the ASEAN nations in southeast Asia, after Myanmar and Thailand, with a 0.1% adult prevalence rate, 130,000 HIV/AIDS cases and 2400deaths. In Jakarta it is estimated that 17% of prostitutes have contracted HIV/AIDS; in some parts of Papua, it is thought that the infection rate among village women who are not prostitutes may be as high as 26%. Three other health hazards facing Indonesia in 2004 were dengue fever, hemorrhagic fever and avian influenza. By 2010 there are three malaria regions in Indonesia. The incidence of malaria has declined to 1.96 per1000 in 2010.

Air Quality has been negatively affected in some years. In 1997 and in 2006 there was a southeast Asian haze produced by smoke with an increase in respiratory symptoms such as asthma, upper respiratory infection decreased lung function as well as eye and skin irritation caused mainly by particulate matter.

Indonesia has routine vaccination of children below the age of 5. The vaccines are produced by PT Bio Pharma which has a certificate from the

WHO. These are preferred in countries with a high Moslem population due to fact that they are halal vaccines. PT BIO Farma produces pentavalent vaccine including hepatitis B and haemophilus influenza type B. They are in the third phase of testing a dengue fever vaccine. The 2010 maternal mortality rate per 100,000 births for Indonesia is 240. The under 5 mortality rate per1000 births is 41and the neonatal mortality as a percentage of under 5s mortality is 49

In 2010, an estimated 56% 0f Indonesians mainly state employees, low income earners and those with private coverage have some form of health insurance. It will boost to100% with a system of Universal social health insurance coverage in place by 2014. The aim is that everybody doesn't have to pay when they are hospitalized in basic/class-3 hospital beds.

HEALTH CARE IN INDIA

Health care facilities and personnel increased substantially between the early 1950s and early 1980s but because of fast population growth the number of licensed medical practitioners per 10,000 individuals had fallen by the late 1980s to three per 10,000 individuals from a level of four in1981. In 1991 there were approximately ten hospital beds per 10,000 individuals. Primary health centers are the cornerstone of the rural healthcare system. By 1991, India had about 22,400 primary health care centers, 11,200 hospitals and 22,400 dispensaries. These facilities are part of a tiered health care system that funnels more difficult cases into the urban hospitals. Primary health centers and subcenters rely on trained paramedics to meet most of the needs. Main problems of these centers is the emphasis on preventive work and a reluctance of staff to work in the rural areas.

According to data provided in 1989 the total number of hospitals for all states and territories was 10,157. In 1991 there was a total 811,000 hospital and health care facilities beds. The geographical distribution of hospitals varied according to local socioeconomic conditions. In India's most populous state, Uttar Pradesh with a 1991 population of more than 139 million there were 735 hospitals. In Kerala with a 1991 population of 29 million there were 2053 hospitals in an area 1/7 the size of Uttar Pradesh. Of the 7,300 hospitals, nearly 4000 were owned and managed by central, state or local governments. Another 2000, owned and managed by charitable trusts received partial support from the government and the remaining 1300 hospitals many of which are relatively small are owned and managed by the private sector. State of the art medical equipment are pretty much confined to urban centers. A network of regional cancer centers was being established in the early 1990s in major hospitals and were part of government medical colleges. By 1992 twenty-two such centers were in operation. Most of the 1,300 private hospitals lacked sophisticated medical facilities. In 1992 only 12% possessed state of the art equipment for the diagnosis and treatment of all major diseases., including cancer.

By the late 1980s there were approximately 128 medical colleges They accepted a combined annual class of 14,166 students. Data for 1987 show that there were 320,000 registered medical practitioners and 219,300 registered nurses. Various studies show that in both urban and rural areas people preferred to pay and seek the more sophisticated services provided by private physicians rather than use free treatment at public health centers.

Indigenous or traditional medical practitioners continue to practice throughout the country. The two main forms of traditional medicine are 'ayurvedic' system which deals with causes, symptoms, diagnosis, and treatment based on all aspects of well-being (mental, physical and spiritual): and the "Unani' an herbal medical practice. These professions are frequently hereditary. A variety of institutions offer training in indigenous medicine. In the early 1990s there were ninety-eight 'ayurvedic' colleges and seventeen 'unani' colleges.

India is a land of many health problems. Nutrition and the standard of living are very poor though there are signs of improvement as the economy grows. The National Health Policy was endorsed by the parliament of India in 1983 updated in2002. The Indian health care industry is seen to be growing at a rapid pace and is expected to become a US$280 billion industry by 2020. Rising income levels and a growing elderly population are all factors driving this growth. Changing demographics, as well as a shift from chronic to lifestyle disease has led to increased spending on health care delivery. In order to meet manpower shortages and reach world standards India would require investments of up to $20 billion over the next 5 years

Healthcare Issues: Malnutrition ranks high. Approximately 1.72 million children die each year before turning one. The under five and infant mortality rate have been declining. However reduced funding for immunization leaves only 43.5% of the young fully immunized. Shortages of healthcare providers, poor intra-partum and newborn care, diarrheal diseases and acute respiratory infections also contribute to the high infant mortality rate.

Diseases: Diseases such as dengue fever, hepatitis, tuberculosis, malaria, and pneumonia are prevalent and continue as persistent problems because of increased resistance to drugs. India now has a totally resistant form of tuberculosis India ranks third amongst countries with HIV infections. Diarrheal diseases are the primary causes of early childhood mortality and all can be attributed to poor sanitation and unsafe drinking water. However in 2012 India was free of polio. Indians are also at high risk for atherosclerosis and coronary heart disease for unknown reasons.

POOR SANITATION: More than 122million households have no toilets and 33% lack access to latrines. Over 50% of the population defecates in the open. This is higher than Bangladesh, Brazil and China. Although 211 million people gained access to improved sanitation from 1990-2008 only 31% uses them. Only 11% of the Indian rural population dispose of child stools safely whereas 80% leave their stools in the open or throw them in the garbage. All of these practices lead to parasitic and bacterial infections

Inadequate safe drinking water: Access to protected sources of drinking water has improved from 68% to 88% of the population in 2008. However, only 26% of the slum population has access to safe drinking water and only 25% of the total population has safe drinking water on the premises. This problem is exacerbated by falling levels of ground water, caused mainly by increased extraction for irrigation. Insufficient protection of their water supplies and sources of water allow ground pollution with excessive arsenic and fluoride in the drinking water.

HEALTH IN THAILAND

Thailand has a successful history of healthcare development according to the World Health Organization. Life expectancy at birth is seventy years. Ninety-eight percent have access to improved drinking water, and ninety-six per-cent have adequate sanitation. A system for providing universal healthcare for Thai nationals has been established since 2002. Health and medical care has been overseen by the ministry of Public Health, along with several other non-ministerial government agencies, with total national expenditure on health amounting to 4.3% of GDP in 2009. Although HIV/AIDS, tuberculosis, malaria, and other infectious diseases remain serious public health issues, non communicable diseases and injuries have also become important causes of morbidity and mortality.

Health Indices: (data from 2009) According to the World Health Organization's Global Health Observatory life expectancy at birth in Thailand is 66years for males and 74 for females. Under 5 mortality rate is 14 per 1000 live births. Maternal mortality is 48 per 100,000 live births. Prevalence of HIV is 13 per 1000 adults and prevalence of tuberculosis is 189 per 100,000 population. Years of life lost was 24% from communicable Disease, 55% from non-communicable disease 22% from injuries.

In 2009, annual spending on health care amounted to 345 dollars per person. Total expenditures represented about 4.3 %of GDP and of this amount 75.8% came from public sources and 24% from private sources. Physician density was 2. 98 per 10,000 in2004 with 22 beds per 100,000 population in 2002.

Improved drinking water sources was available to 98% of the population and 96% of the population were using improved sanitation facilities. Data for utilization of health services in 2008 included contraception, attended births, measles immunization, and treatment of smear positive tuberculosis.

The majority of health care services in Thailand is delivered by the public sector which includes 1002 hospitals and 9,765 health stations. Universal health care is provided through three programs: the civil service welfare system for civil servants and their families, Social Security for private employees, and the Universal Coverage Scheme theoretically available to all other Thai nationals. Private hospitals are participants in these programs but most are financed by patient self-payment and private insurance.

The Ministry of Public Health oversees national health policy and also operates most government health facilities. The National Health Security Office allocates funding through the Universal Coverage program. Other health related government agencies include the Health System Research Institute, Thai Health Promotion Foundation, National Health Commission Office and the Emergency Medical Institute of Thailand. The Ministry of Public Health still controls most aspects of health care.

Thailand introduced universal coverage reforms in 2001, becoming one of only a handful of lower-middle income countries to do so. Means-tested health care for low income households was replaced by a new and more comprehensive insurance scheme, originally known as the 30 baht project in line with the small copayment charged for treatment. People joining the scheme receive a gold card which allows them to access services in their health district and if necessary be referred for specialist treatment. The bulk of finance comes from public revenue., with funding allocated to Contracting Units for Primary Care annually on a population basis. According to the WHO, 65% of Thailand's health care expenditure in2004 came from the government while 35% came from private sources. The reforms have proved popular with the poorer Thais, especially in the rural areas, and survived the change of government after the 2006 military coup. Then the public health minister abolished the 30 baht co-payment and made the UC scheme free.

HOSPITALS IN THAILAND; Most hospitals in Thailand are operated by the ministry of Public Health. Private hospitals are regulated by the Medical registration Division under the MOPH's Department of health Service Support following the 'Sanatorium act'. Other government units and public organizations also operate hospitals, including the military, universities, local governments, and the Red Cross. As of 2010 there are 1002 public hospitals and 316 registered private hospitals.

Provincial hospitals operated by the MOPH's Office of the permanent Secretary are classified as follows;

- Regional hospitals are located in province centers, have a capacity of at least 500 beds and have a comprehensive set of specialists on staff.
- General hospitals are located in province capitals or major districts and have a capacity of 200 to 500 beds

- Community hospitals are located in the district level and further classified by size

   Large community hospitals have a capacity of 90 to 150 beds
   Medium community hospitals have a capacity of 60 beds
   Small community hospitals have a capacity of 10 to 30 beds

While all three types of hospitals serve the local population, community hospitals are usually limited to providing primary care, while referring patients in need of more advanced or specialized care to general or regional hospitals. Private hospitals with less than 30 beds are officially termed 'health centers'

Important public Health Issues: Infectious Disease, most notably HIV/AIDS and tuberculosis remain serious public health problems. Non-communicable disease and injuries have become important causes of morbidity and mortality. Major infectious diseases in Thailand include diarrhea, hepatitis, dengue fever, malaria, encephalitis, rabies and leptospirosis. HIV/AIDS is a serious problem in Thailand. Prevalence has decreased to an estimated 1.5% of all persons aged 15 to 49 years. It was also reported that 58,000 adults and children had died from AIDS since 1984. The government has funded a retroviral drug program and as of 2006 more than 80,000 HIV/AIDS patients had received such drugs.

Bangkok hospitals cater to foreign patients and are well equipped. The price of treatment is fixed and you will be told before treatment how much it costs and be asked to pay in advance. Room and nursing costs are about 3,000-6,000 baht a day. Outpatient treatment is well organized, about 700-1000 baht range and does not require payment in advance.

Ambulance transportation is not readily available. Stay near a hospital and have money to pay up front if you need a hospital bed.

HEALTH CARE SYSTEM IN JAPAN

The health care system in Japan provides the usual examinations, prenatal care, and infectious disease control with the patient accepting responsibility for 30% of these costs while the government pays the remaining 70%. Payment for personal medical service is offered through a universal health care insurance system that provides relative equality of access with fees set by a government committee. People without insurance through employers can participate in a national health insurance program administered by local governments. Patients are free to select physicians or facilities of their choice and cannot be denied coverage. Hospitals by law must be run as non-profit and be managed by physicians. For-profit corporations are not allowed to own or operate hospitals. Clinics must be operated and owned by physicians.

Since 1961 Japan has provided universal health coverage which allows virtually all to access preventive, curative, and rehabilitative services at an affordable cost. The patients accept responsibility for 10%, 20%, or 30% of these costs while the government pays the remaining. People without insurance through employers can participate in a national health insurance program administered by local governments. Patients are free to select physicians or facilities of their choice.

COST: In 2008, Japan spent about 8.5% of the nations gross domestic product (GDP) or US$2,873 per capita on health which ranked 20th among Organization for Economic Co-operation Development (OECD) countries. It was less than an average 9.6% across OECD countries in 2009, and about half as much as that in the US. The government has well controlled costs over decades by using the nationally uniform fee schedule for reimbursement. Fees for all health care are set every two years by negotiations between the health ministry and physicians. The negotiations determine the fee for every medical procedure and medication and fees are identical across the country. If physicians try to game the system by ordering more procedures to generate income the government may lower the fees at the next round of fee setting. For example the fee for MRI was lowered 35% in 2002 by the government. Japan has had catastrophic coverage since 1973. Once monthly co-pay reaches the cap, no more copayment is required. The monthly copayment amount is tiered into three levels according to income and age.

QUALITY: People in Japan have the longest life expectancy at birth in the world. Life expectancy at birth was 83 years in 2009 This was achieved through a reduction in mortality rates secondary to communicable diseases in the 50s and 60s as well as a large reduction in stroke mortality rates.

In 2008 acute care beds per 1000 total population was 8.1 which was higher than other OECD countries, such as the US (2.7). 34% of patients were admitted to the hospital for longer than 30 days even in beds that were classified as acute care.

In 2008 there were 2.2 practicing phsycians per 1000 population which was almost the same as that in the US (2.4), and the number of practicing nurses was 9.5 which was a little lower than that in the US(10.8) and almost the same as that in the UK (9.5) or in Canada (9.2) Physicians and nurses are licensed for life with no requirement for license renewal, continuing medical or nursing education and no peer or utilization review. OECD data puts generalists and specialists together for Japan because these two are not officially differentiated. Traditionally physicians were trained to become subspecialist but once they completed training only a few continued to practice as a subspecialist and the rest left the large hospitals to practice in small community hospitals or open their own clinics without any formal retraining as a generalist.

In Japan, services are provided either through regional/national public hospitals or through private hospitals / clinics and patients have access to any facility though hospitals tend to charge higher for those without a referral. Japanese patients favor medical technology such as CT scan and MRI and they receive MRI at a per capita 8 times higher than the British and twice the amount of the Americans. Japan has about 3 times as many hospitals per capita as the US and on average people visit the hospital more than 4 times as often as the average American. The problem has become a wide concern in Japan, particularly in Tokyo. A report that more than 14,000 emergency patients were rejected at least three times by hospitals in Japan before getting treatment in 2007 according to the government survey for that year, got a lot of attention when it was released in 2009, and around this time there were several incidents reported in the Tokyo area such as an elderly man who was turned away by 14 hospitals before dying 90 minutes after being finally admitted. And a case of a pregnant woman complaining of severe headache being refused admission to seven Tokyo hospitals and later dying of an undiagnosed brain hemorrhage after giving birth.

INSURANCE; Health insurance is in general mandatory for residents of Japan though there is no penalty on individuals who choose not to comply and around 10% of the population does not enroll. There are a total of eight insurance systems in Japan. They can be divided into two categories, Employees Health Insurance and National Health Insurance. Employees Health Insurance is broken down to the following systems

- * Union Managed Health Insurance
- * Government Managed Health Insurance
- * Seaman's Insurance
- * National Public Workers Mutual Aid Association Insurance
- * Local Public Workers Mutual Aid Association Insurance

National Health Insurance is generally reserved for self-employed people and students, whereas social insurance is normally for corporate employees. National Health Insurance can be broken down into

- * National Health Insurance for each city, town or village
- * National Health Insurance Union

Public health insurance covers most citizens /residents and the system pays 70% or more of medical and prescription drug costs with the remainder being covered by the patient. The monthly insurance premium is per household and scaled to annual income. Supplementary private health insurance is available only to cover the co-payments or non-covered costs, and usually makes a fixed payment per days in hospital or per surgery performed rather than actual expenditure.

HISTORY OF HEALTH CARE IN JAPAN: The beginning of the Japanese Health Care System began in 1927 when the first Employee Health Insurance Plan was created. In 1961, Japan achieved universal health insurance coverage and almost everyone became insured. However the co-payment rates differed greatly. While those who enrolled in Employees Health Insurance needed to pay only a nominal amount at the first physician visit, their dependents and those who enrolled in National Health Insurance had to pay 50% of the fee schedule price for all services and medications. From 1961 to 1982 this 50% co-payment rate was gradually lowered to 30%. Since 1983 all elderly persons have been covered by government sponsored insurance.

By the early 1990s there were more than 1000 mental hospitals, 8700 general hospitals, and 1000 comprehensive hospitals with a total capacity of 1.5 million beds. Hospitals provided both out-patient and in-patient care. In addition, 79000 clinics offered primarily out-patient services and there were 48,000 dental clinics. Most physicians and hospitals sold medication directly to the patient but there were 36,000 pharmacies where patients could purchase medications. National health expenditures rose from about 1 trillion yen in 1965 to nearly 20 trillion yen in1989, or from slightly more than 5% to more than 6% of Japan's national income. The system has been troubled with excessive paperwork, assembly-line care for out-patients (few facilities made appointments), over-medication, and abuse of the system because of apparent low out-of-pocket expense to patients. Another problem is an uneven distribution of health personnel with rural areas favored over cities.

In the early 1900s, there were nearly 191,000 physicians, 66,800 dentists, 333,000 nurses, plus 200,000 people licensed to practice massage, acupuncture, moxibustion, and other East Asian therapeutic methods.

The Japanese have been described as the healthiest group on the planet. Whether this is true or not is not proven but because of universal health care the Japanese visit a doctor nearly 14 times a year which is about four times as often as Americans. Japan's suicide rate is high compared to the USA and it was reported that more than 30,000 people had killed themselves every year for the past decade.

Other problems prominent in Japanese society are smoking and alcohol. It is believed smoking contributes or is the cause of 100,000 deaths per year. It is also estimated that the social cost of excessive drinking of alcoholic beverages in Japan runs to 4.15 trillion yen per year. Chinese traditional medicine and herbal medicine is still available but modern western style medicine is the standard and is widely practiced and sought.

AIDS: AIDS cases are relatively small in number by world standards but are of great concern to Public Health officials. By 1991 there were 553 cases and by 1992 this had risen to 2077. Most Japanese are not concerned with acquiring the disease themselves but the government has established committees sympathetic to the plight of hemophiliacs as well as the heterosexual population mandating AIDS education and advising testing for the general public without targeting specific groups.

Radiation effects from Fukushima Daiichi nuclear disaster: Mention must be made of the Fukushima nuclear disaster on 11 march 2011. The radioactivity released, the number of people exposed to harmful radiation, the effects of exposed food such as rice and fish, water, the residual radiation, and certainly the significant psychological effects from fear and worry for self, family and the nation will be studied for years to come. The results thus far do not indicate severe damage except for a very few who were exposed at the site of the reactor. Japanese officials initially assessed the accident as a level 4 on the international Nuclear Event Scale. The level was eventually raised to a 7. The government estimates the total amount of radio activity released into the atmosphere was approximately one-tenth as much as was released during the Chernobyl disaster. A few of the plant's workers were severely injured or killed by the earthquake there were no immediate deaths due to direct radiation exposure, but at least six workers have exceeded lifetime legal limits for radiation and more than 300 have received significant radiation doses. Decontamination will take decades. Future cancer deaths due to accumulated radiation exposure in the population living near have been estimated between 100 and 1000.

HEALTHCARE IN DENMARK

Healthcare in Denmark is largely financed through local (county and municipal) taxation with integrated funding and provision of health care at the local county level.

Denmark spends 9.8 % of GDP on healthcare. The life expectancy in Denmark is 78.6 years. There is one doctor for every 294 persons in Denmark

PRIMARY CARE: Most primary care in Denmark is provided by general practitioners, who are paid on a combined capitation and fee-for-service basis in a similar way to those in the United Kingdom. The counties determine the number and location of general practitioners, and their fees and working conditions are negotiated centrally between the physician's union and the government. The municipal health services provide health visitors, home nurses and school health care,

SECONDARY CARE: Hospital care is mainly provided by hospitals owned and run by the county. (or the Copenhagen Hospital Corporation in the Copenhagen area) This is similar to the model in other Scandinavian countries. There are a few private hospital providers and they account for less than 1% of hospital beds.

CENTRAL GOVERNMENT ROLE: The central government plays a relatively limited role in health care in Denmark. Its main functions are to regulate, coordinate, and provide advice and its main responsibilities are to establishing goals for national health policy, determining national health legislation, formulating regulation, promoting cooperation between different health care actors, providing guidelines for the health sector, providing health and health-care related information, promoting quality and tackling patient complaints.

DENMARK—HEALTH Denmark's health care system has retained the same basic structure since the early 1970s. The administration of hospitals and personnel is dealt with by the Ministry of the Interior, while primary care facilities, health insurance, and community care are the primary responsibility of the Ministry of Social Affairs. Anyone can go to a physician for no fee and the public health system entitles each Dane to his /her own doctor. Expert medical/surgical aid is available, with a qualified nursing staff. Costs are borne by public authority, but high taxes contribute to these costs. As of 1999 there were an estimated 3-4 physicians and 4-5 hospital beds per 1000 people. The number of hospital beds, like that in other EU countries has undergone a major decline since 1980 from around 40,000 to about 23,000 in 1998/99. Deinstitutionalization of psychiatric patients has contributed significantly to this trend. The ratio of doctors to population, by contrast, has increased during this period.

The total fertility rate in 2000 (Denmark) was 1.7 while the maternal mortality rate was 10 per 100,000 live births as of 1998. Cardiovascular disease and cancer were the leading causes of death. Denmark's cancer rate was the highest in the European Union. In1999, the number of people living with HIV/AIDS was estimated at 4300 and deaths that year from AIDS were estimated at less than100. There were only 12 reported cases of tuberculosis.

Danish citizens may choose between two systems of primary care: medical care provided free of charge by a doctor whom the individual chooses for a year and by those specialists to whom the doctor refers the patient; or complete freedom of choice of any physician or specialist at any time, with state reimbursement of about 2/3of the cost for medical bills paid directly by the patient. Most Danes opt for the former All patients receive subsidies on pharmaceuticals and vital drugs; all patients must pay a share of dental bills. As of 1999, total health care expenditure was estimated at 8.4%of GDP.

HEALTH IN BRAZIL

Health care in Brazil is provided by both private and government institutions. The Minister for Health and Ageing administers national health policy. Primary health care remains the responsibility of the federal government elements of which (such as operation of hospitals) are overseen by individual states. Public health care is provided to all Brazilian permanent residents, and foreigners in Brazilian territory and is free at the point of need (being paid for from general taxation). The country is the home of several of the international health organizations, such as the Latin American and Caribbean Center on Health Sciences Information, and the Edumed Institute for Education in Medicine and Health. Life expectancy for females is 77.3; for males 69.7; Infant mortality 22.58; fertility 1.76; childhood mortality about 2.51% reaching 3.77% in the northeast region; motherhood mortality about 73.1 deaths per 100.000 born children; non transmissible illness 151.7 deaths per 100,000 inhabitants caused by heart and circulatory disease; cancer causes 72.7 deaths per 100,000 inhabitants; mortality caused by external causes such as violence, suicide, transportation 71.7 per 100,000. In 2002 Brazil accounted for 40% of malaria cases in the Americas, 99% of these in the Amazon region. Brazil lags behind countries such as Japan, Switzerland, Iceland, Australia, France, Italy where the life expectancy is already over 81.

Infant Mortality (Brazil): There has been a significant decline in infant mortality rates over the last 30 years. Despite this, however mortality rates are still high by international standards. Sanitation, education, and per capita income are the most explanatory factors of poor child health in Brazil. UNICEF report shows a rising rate of survival for Brazilian children under the age of five. UNICEF says that out of a total 195 countries Brazil is among the 25 nations with the best improvement in survival rates for children under the age of five. The report shows that Brazil's infant mortality rate for live births in 2008 was 22 per thousand, a drop of 61%since 1990. Mortality rates for children at one year of age was 18 per thousand, a reduction of 60%. The study went onto show that malnutrition among children less than 2 years of age in the period 2000 and 2008 fell by 77%. UNICEF called the numbers an enormous victory for brazil though poverty remains a major problem and much still needs to be done.

Health care system: The national health policy is based on the Federal Constitution of 1988, which sets out the principles and directives for the delivery of health care in the country through the Unified Health System (SUS). Under the constitution, the activities of the federal government are to be based on multiyear plans approved by the national congress for four year periods. The current legal provisions governing the operation of the health system instituted in 1996 seek to shift responsibility for administration of the SUS to municipal governments with technical and financial cooperation from the federal government and states. Another regionalization initiative is the creation of health consortia which pools the resources of several neighboring municipalities.

INDIVIDUAL HEALTH CARE SERVICES (Brazil); In 1999, 66% of the country's 7806 hospitals, and 70% of its 485,000 hospital beds and 87% of its 723 specialized hospitals belonged to the private sector. In the area of diagnostic support 95% of the 7,318 establishments were also private. 73% of the 41,000 ambulatory care facilities were operated by the public sector. An estimated 25% of the population is covered by at least one form of health insurance. 75% of the insurance plans are offered by commercial operators.

National health expenditure amounted to 7.9% of GDP. Of that total, public spending accounted for 42.2% and private expenditure accounted for 58.8 %.

HUMAN RESOURCE In 1999, the country had 237,000 physicians, 145,000 dentists, 77,000 nurses, 26,000 dietitions, and 56,000 veterinarians.

EMERGENCY SERVICES Brazilian emergency medical service is locally called the SAMU (mobile emergency attendance service). Brazil still lacks a consistent standard of care. Pre-hospital emergency medical services use a combination of basic ambulances staffed by technicians and some advanced units may have a physician on board. The dispatch center physician determines whether the call merits an emergency transport. No universal phone number exists for emergency calls. Portaria 2048 calls upon the entire health care system to improve emergency care in order to address the increasing number of victims resulting from road traffic accidents and violence, as well as the overcrowding of emergency departments. Emergency staff physicians come from a variety of backgrounds often as a supplement to private practice. Since 50% of medical school graduates do not get residency positions these new physicians look for work in the emergency departments. In the larger tertiary hospitals the ED is divided into main specialty areas such as internal medicine, surgery, psychiatry, pediatrics etc. In the non tertiary care centers which make up the majority of hospitals, emergency department physicians are largely under-trained, underpaid, and overstressed by their working conditions. There is a very large need for improvement in the emergency care system.

A current plan in action in Brazil is the CATCH plan. (Commission for the Advancement of Technology for Communications and Health). Funding is provided by the WHO, ITU, and voluntary countries and benefactors for existing and future projects.

HEALTH CARE IN ARGENTINA

Argentina's health care system is composed of three sectors: the public sector, financed through taxes; the private sector, financed through voluntary insurance schemes; and the social sector, financed through obligatory insurance schemes. The Ministry of Health and Social Action (MSAS) oversees all three subsectors of the health care system and is responsible for setting of regulation.

HEALTH CARE OBRAS SOCIALES (Argentina)

The public sector is funded and managed by Obras Sociales, umbrella organizations for Argentine worker's unions. There are over 300 Obras Sociales in Argentina, each chapter being organized according to the occupation of the beneficiary. These organizations vary greatly in quality and effectiveness. The top 30 chapters hold 73% of the beneficiaries and 75% of resources for health care. MSAS has established a Solidarity Redistribution Fund to try to address these beneficiary inequities. Only workers employed in the formal sector are covered under Obras Sociales insurance schemes and after Argentina's economic crises of 2001, the number of those covered under these schemes fell slightly (as unemployment increased and employment in the formal sector rose). In 1999 there were 8.9 million beneficiaries covered by Obras Sociales.

PRIVATE SECTOR (Argentina)

The private health care sector in Argentina is characterized by great heterogeneity and is made up of a great number of fragmented facilities and small networks; it consists of over 200 organizations and covers approximately 2 million Argentines. Private insurance often overlaps with other forms of health care coverage thus it is difficult to estimate the degree to which beneficiaries are dependent on the public and private sectors. According to a 2000 report by the IRBC, foreign competition has increased in Argentina's private sector, with Swiss, American, and other Latin American health care providers entering the market. In recent years this has been accompanied by little formal regulation.

THE PUBLIC SYSTEM (Argentina)

The Public System is highly decentralized to the provincial level; often primary care is even under the purview of local townships. In 2001 the number of Argentines relying on public services has seen an increase. According to 2000 figures, 37.4% of Argentines had no health insurance, 48.8% were covered under Obras Sociales, 8.6% had private insurance, and 3.8% were covered by both Obras Sociales and private insurance. There are over 9 million people who are covered by public health care. However this not public healthcare as you might typically think of it. It is run by an umbrella of union organizations. This means that instead of the government controlling your healthcare it will be controlled by your union. Right now you have to be employed and paying dues to one of the union organizations to be covered. It will also cover your dependents. This can cause problems if you are unemployed

The public system of health care within Argentina is described in one article as a big mess and many people using these services are not getting the best treatment. There are not enough doctors and there is a shortage of staff in the hospitals. This leads to longer waits for those who are ill. Equipment is often inadequate, getting a simple x-ray and the needed medication can be difficult if you are not in a major city.

HEALTHCARE IN CHILE

All workers and pensioners are mandated to pay 7% of their income for healthcare insurance (the poorest pensioners are exempt from this payment). Workers who choose not to join an Isapre are automatically covered by Fonasa. Fonasa also covers unemployed people receiving unemployment benefits, uninsured pregnant women, insured worker's dependent family, people with mental or physical disability and people who are considered poor or indigent.

Fonasa beneficiares may seek attention at public or private facilities. When choosing public Health facilities the cost is free for people older than 60, people without income or with disabilities and for workers earning less than one minimum wage (MW), or less than 1.46 minimum wage (MW) if they have three or more dependents to take care of. Workers earning between one and 1.46MW and having less than two dependents, or earning more than 1.46MWand having three or more dependents pay 10% of the costs. Workers earning more than 1.46MW pay 20% of costs if they have two or less dependents to look after.

Workers covered by Fonasa may seek attention in the private sector if the private health facility or health professional is associated with Fonasa in one of three price levels. The higher the level the more expensive the cost for the worker. The level of protection offered by the Isapre system depends on the worker's income and their medical risk, estimated by their age, sex, family medical history etc. Chile's Constitutional court declared risk determination based on sex and age to be unconstitutional. Isapre participants pay on average 9.2% of their income toward health insurance. The additional paid over the required 7% is voluntary and is paid to increase the benefits available. Almost 60% of payers are in the top two quintiles of income while only 7% are in the bottom quintiles. Isapres often use networks of providers to offer discounted benefits. They also offer shorter time waiting for services. Fonasa, on the other hand uses lower cost public hospitals, and can include a broader benefit package for the same cost. The trade-off is quicker accessibility to services.

Over 50% of the public sector health budget is raised through taxation—this goes to the public social security system and the Fonasa plans to help cover expenses. Isapres cover all expenses using only the contributions of members.

AUGE Plan: there are a number of high mortality pathological conditions(currently69) that have special guarantees for both Isapre and Fonasa affiliates. The 'AUGE' or 'GES plan includes four guarantees in relation to these illnesses

* Access: individuals will be able to get attention from a network of providers near their place of residence
* Opportunity: there is a maximum pre-established time limit to get attention (both initial attention and after the diagnosis)
* Quality: services will follow technical requirement standards that will be established based on medical evidence
* Financial coverage: Payment to providers cannot be an obstacle to attention. There will be a maximum copayment of 20% of the cost, with the total not to exceed one month of income for the family in a year.

			Beneficiares by December 2009
System	Affiliates	%	
FONASA	12,504,226	73.49	
Isapre	2,705,917	15.90	
TOTAL POP.	17,014,491	100	

Health Care in General: Healthcare in Chile is very advanced and state-of-the-art on the high end. The national health care system (FONASA) provides basic medical service and coverage to all levels of society. Quality is better at private clinics and hospitals around Chile, though even the most expensive private clinics are relatively affordable (at least by US standards). Doctors are well trained and professional. Hospitals are generally run as professional businesses with national regulation of standards that meet or exceed international standards of care. Chile tends to rank well on international benchmarks comparing metrics such as life expectancy at birth or infant mortality.

INSURANCE: Medical care is offered through two systems: FONASA (government) and ISAPRES (private)

DOCTORS: Chile does not have a system of Primary Care or having a local GP as the norm, like other countries. General Practitioners can be relatively rare as most doctors specialize if they can. The type of family doctor who might be the first point of contact for medical concerns is not a concept well known in Chile as it is in other countries, but they do exist. You do not need a referral to see a specialist, so many go directly to the specialist. To see a doctor you will need to buy a bono in advance. If you have insurance (FONASA) or ISAPRE) then you will pay the co-pay amount. In some consults you can do this on the spot, electronically, but in others you will need to have bought your bono in advance. For example, if you have a Colmena as your Isapre you will go to Colmena before your appointment and buy a bono. You can pay cash and then get reimbursed afterwards. Usually you will pay less if you buy in advance. If you do not have insurance, you will pay as a "Particular". The cost varies depending on the doctor. A general practitioner in Antofagasta costs $15,000 particular. If the doctor orders blood tests or X-rays, then you will be given a script. You will need to buy a bono. Your ISAPRE will need the doctors script in order to sell you a bono. ISAPRESs have different agreement s with different testing centers. A blood test in one place may cost you nothing (costo zero) and down the road the same test is $15,000.

For blood tests, they might all end up at the same lab, but depending on where the blood is drawn the cost is different. Again with your script, you will be able to pay privately if you have no health insurance. You will pick up your results and then will need to go back and see your doctor again if you need them interpreted. There is no communication back to your doctor about your results

LICENCIA MEDICA: If you are employed in Chile and you are sick for even one day, you will need to present a Medical Certificate or "Licencia Medica". Universities, schools and even some day care centers also require them for absence. A Licencia for 3 days or less is not paid for.

A Licencia for more than 3 days, the first 3 days are not paid for but the remaining days are. A Licencia for for 11 days or more is paid for all days. Sick days covered are paid by your ISAPRE.

HOSPITALS: One of the best hospitals in Chile is Clinica Alemanas in Santiago. Other Clinica Alemanas can be found in most major cities in Chile and also are excellent. Clinica Alemanas in Santiago is recognized as one of the best and most advanced hospitals in the country. Another reputed hospital in Santiago is Clinica Las Condes.

In Chile a 'hospital' is public. A 'Clinica' is a private hospital. Treatment and surroundings will be better in a Clinica. Both may run emergency departments however waiting times are determined by the gravity of the problem. Some ERs do attend by order of arrival. In the 'clinica' you will be asked to pay. If you are admitted to a hospital via the ER you will be asked to pay or at least sign a 'pagare' or a guarantee that you will pay when the bill comes in and details about your health insurance.

Pharmacies: Drug prices may be considered low by some expatriates and to others who have come from highly subsidized systems, very high. Many pharmacies are open 24 hours a day. They offer free or cheap home deliveries in the biggest cities. Drugs that are commonly sold over-the-counter in the USA are often kept behind the counter at pharmacies in Chile. Many drugs that require a prescription in the USA, such as insulin, do not require a prescription in Chile.

HEALTHCARE IN SOUTH AFRICA

In South Africa, parallel private and public systems exist. The public system serves the vast majority of the population, but is chronically under-funded and under-staffed.

The wealthiest 20% of the population uses the private system and are far better served. In 2005, South Africa spent 8.7% of GDP on health care, or $ 437 per capita. Of that approximately 42% was government expenditure. About 79% of doctors work in the private sector.

HIV/AIDS in SOUTH AFRICA: HIV and AIDS in South Africa are major health concerns, and about 5.5 million people are thought to be living with the virus in South Africa. South Africa has more people with HIV/AIDS than any other country. The South African National HIV Survey estimated that 10.8% of all South Africans over 2 years old were living with HIV in 2005. There is an average of almost 1,000 deaths of AIDS a day in South Africa.

Other infectious diseases prevalent in South Africa include: Bacterial diarrhea, Typhoid Fever, and Hepatitis A. These infectious diseases are generally caused when the food or water consumed by an individual has been exposed to fecal material. South Africa is an under-developed nation and because of this the sanitation facility access in urban areas is 16% unimproved while in rural areas the sanitation facility access is 35% unimproved.

UPFS: The public sector uses a Uniform Patient Fee Schedule as a guide to billing for services. This is being used in all the provinces of South Africa, although in Western Cape, Kwa-Zulu Natal and Eastern Cape it is being implemented on a phased schedule. It groups patients into three categories: full paying patients; fully subsidized patients and partially subsidized patients. There are also specified occasions in which services are free of cost.

ANTIRETROVIRAL TREATMENT: Because of its many cases of HIV/AIDS among citizens (about 5.6 million in 2009) South Africa has been working to create a program to distribute anti-retroviral therapy treatment, which has been generally limited in low economic countries. In 2003 the operational Plan for comprehensive HIV and AIDS care, management, and treatment was approved. This was accompanied by a National Strategic Plan for 2007-2011. According to the World Health Organization. about 37% of infected individuals were receiving treatment at the end of 2009. It wasn't until 2009 that the South African National Aids Council urged the government to raise the treatment threshold to be within World Health Organization guidelines. The latest anti-retroviral treatment guidelines, released in February 2010 continue to fall short of these recommendations. In the beginning of 2010 the government promised to treat all HIV-positive children with anti-retroviral therapy but some studies show a lack of concern for children in many hospitals. In 2009 a little over 50% of children in need of antiretroviral therapy were receiving it. Only 37% of those considered in need of anti-retroviral therapy are receiving it.

One of the controversies surrounding the distribution of anti-retroviral drugs is the use of generic drugs. When an effective drug became available in1996 only economically rich countries could afford it at a price of $10,000-$15,000 per year. In 2000 generic anti-retroviral treatments started being produced and sold at a much cheaper cost. Needing to compete with these prices, the big brand companies were forced to lower their prices. The anti-retroviral treatment can now be purchased as low as eighty-eight dollars per person per year.

HEALTHCARE PROVISION IN THE POSTWAR PERIOD

Following the end of the Second World War, South Africa saw a rapid growth in the coverage by private insurance though this mainly benefited the middle class white population. From 1945 to 1960 the percentage of whites covered by health insurance grew from 48% to 80% of that population. Virtually the entire white population had shifted away from the free health services provided by the government by 1960, although 95% of non-whites remained reliant on the public sector for treatment. Membership in health insurance schemes was compulsory for white South Africans because membership was a condition of employment and virtually all whites were employed. Pensioner members of many health insurance schemes received the same medical benefits as other members of these schemes, but free of cost. Since coming to power in 1994, the African National Congress (ANC) has implemented a number of measures to combat health inequality in South Africa. These have included the introduction of free health care in 1994 for all children under the age of six together with pregnant and breast feeding women making use of public sector health facilities and the extension of free hospital care to children older than six with moderate and severe disabilities.

NHI (NATIONAL HEALTH INSURANCE. The current South African government is working to establish a national health insurance (NHI) system out of concern for discrepancies within the national health care system, such as unequal access to healthcare amongst different socio-economic groups. Although the details and outline of the proposal have yet to be released, it seeks to find ways to make health care more available to those who can't afford it or whose situation prevents them from attaining the services they need. Because the discrepancy of money spent in the private sector (which serves the wealthy) and then spent in the public sector (which serves the majority of the population) the total population does not have health care coverage, most of whom are low or middle class, and perhaps need it more. The NHI proposes a single National Health Insurance Fund (NHIF) for health insurance. This fund is expected to draw its revenue from general taxes and some sort of health insurance contribution. Those receiving health care from both public and private sectors will be mandated to contribute through taxes to the NHIF. The ANC hopes that the NHI plan will work to pay for health care costs for those who cannot pay. Currently the vast majority of health funds comes from individual contributions coming from upper class patients paying directly for care in the private sector. The NHI proposes that health care fund revenues be shifted from these individual contributions to a general tax revenue.

MATERNAL AND CHILD HEALTHCARE: In June 2011 the United Nations released a report on The State of the World's Midwifery. It contained new data on midwifery, newborn and maternal mortality for 58 countries. The 2010 maternal mortality per 100,000 births for South Africa is 410. This is compared with 236.8 in 2008 and 120.7 in 1990. The under 5 mortality rate per 1000 births is 65 and the neonatal mortality as a percentage of under 5's mortality is 30. The aim of this report for South Africa is to reduce child mortality and improve maternal death rates. 1 in 100 is the lifetime risk of death for pregnant women.

Public versus Private. The private sector attracts most of the country's health professionals. Although the state contributes about 40% of all expenditure on health the public health sector is under pressure to deliver services to about 80% of the population. This same discrepancy is seen in drug expenditure per person. The number of private hospitals and clinics continues to grow. Four Years ago there were 161 private hospitals now there are 200. The mining industry provides its own hospitals and has 60 hospitals and clinics around the country. Most health professionals, except nurses work in private hospitals. Public health consumes around 11% of the government's total budget which is allocated and spent by the nine provinces. With less resources and more poor people, cash-strapped provinces like the Eastern Cape face greater health challenges.

HEALTHCARE IN FINLAND

Health care in Finland consists of a highly decentralized, three level publicly funded health care system and a much smaller private health care sector. Although the Ministry of Social Affairs and Health has the highest decision making authority, the municipalities (local government) are responsible for providing health care to their residents. Finland offers its residents universal health care. Health promotion, including prevention of disease has been the main focus of Finnish health care policies for decades. This has resulted in the eradication of certain communicable diseases and improvement in the health of the population. Current challenges in the Finnish health care system are waiting lists in ambulatory care, staff shortages in certain municipalities, the increasing health care expenditures due to an aging population and the increasing cost of the health care technology.

The quality of service in Finnish health care is considered to be good, and according to a survey published by the European Commission in 2000, Finland has the highest number of people satisfied with their hospital care system in the EU: 88% of Finnish respondents were satisfied compared with the EU average of 41.3%

History: Finland's journey to a welfare state has been long and from a very modest start. The history of modern medicine in Finland can be considered to have begun in 1640 when the first University of Finland The Royal Academy of Turku was established. At that time Finland was part of the Swedish empire. The importance of a medical faculty remained low until 1750 when the professor of medicine was the only trained doctor in Finland. Finland had a much lower doctor patient ratio compared to the neighboring countries all the way until the 20th century.

The number of hospitals increased rapidly from the late 19th century. Main reasons for mortality were coronary heart disease for men and cancer of the breast for women. In 1929 a special committee was established to evaluate the situation in health care. It was suggested that municipalities would establish hospitals. These publicly funded hospitals are the base of the current model of modern health care in Finland. The Second World War may have delayed the development but the large number of casualties enhanced the development. In the 1950 Finland had two university hospitals in Helsinki and in Turku. Due to the increased demand and lack of medical doctors more medical faculties and university hospitals were established. During the 20th century Arvo Ylppo made notable contributions to the reduction of infant mortality as well as to nursing education, pharmacy and public awareness.

HEALTH CARE INDICATORS: Finnish health care can be considered good by several indicators. There has been remarkable improvements in life expectancy in Finland over the past few decades. Life expectancy in 2011 is 83 years for women and 75 years for men all of which ranks high on a global scale. In Finland infant mortality and maternal mortality rates are among the lowest in the world. Infant mortality stood at 2.6 deaths per 1000 live births.

In 2009 Finland had 2.7 practicing physicians per 1000 population which was the lowest among the Nordic countries. This can partly be explained by the important role that nurses play for reducing the need for physician consultations. In 2009 there were 9.6 nurses per 1000 population. Finland is successful in particular as regards specialized medical care and the coverage of screenings and vaccinations. Finland has a very comprehensive screening program for breast cancer and a vaccination program that covers 99% of the children for whooping cough and measles.

The most significant public Health problems currently are circulatory diseases, cancer, musculoskeletal diseases and mental health problems. Emerging problems are obesity, chronic lung diseases, and type 2 diabetes. Major causes of death in Finland are cardiovascular diseases, malignant tumors, dementia and Alzheimers disease, respiratory diseases, alcohol related disease and accidental poisoning by alcohol.

Suicide mortality in Finland has generally been one of the, highest in Europe, but it has reduced to 18 per 100,000 in 2005. One reason for this may be the large national suicide prevention project which was carried out between 1986 and 1996.

HIV/AIDS is not a major problem in Finland The prevalence among adult population in 2009 was 0.1%. The countries near Finland have much higher rates due to increased travel. The aging population and the decreased fertility brings new challenges because there will be fewer people to pay for health and social care. It is estimated that the old age dependency ratio in Finland will be the highest of all EU countries in 2025. The total alcohol consumption has risen from 7.6 litres (in1985) to 10 litres of 100% alcohol equivalent per capita in 2010. Although consumption is average to other western countries, binge drinking and intoxication remains characteristic of Finnish drinking habits. Smoking among adults has shown a decline and now the smoking rates among adults in Finland in 2009 is 18.6%. Drug use is not a major public health problem. 3% had used cannabis in the last 12 months.

HEALTH FINANCING: The health care system receives funding from two sources. Municipal financing is based on taxes and is used to provide primary health care services. They also have a right to collect user fees, and receive state subsidies if their tax levy is not adequate for providing the public services required, based on demographic factors in their area. Municipalities fund the health centers on the primary care level and regional hospitals on the secondary level. As municipalities are both the providers and purchasers of the health services it does not make for cost-efficiency. National Health Insurance (NHI) is based on compulsory fees and it is used to fund private health care, occupational health care, outpatient drugs and sickness allowance. Regional and university hospitals are financed by federations of participating municipalities, often using the diagnosis-related group system.

USER FEES: The out of pocket fee amount for a doctor's visit or treatment in the primary health care is set at a maximum of EUR 13.79 and the amount varies from one local authority to another. Hospital out-patients pay 27.40 EUR per consultation; in-patients pay a per diem charge of EUR 32.50. For long-term illness, the charges are based largely on income. Although a vital part of health financing and provision, the current system of user fees is felt to contribute to the inequities in the access to health services among low income residents.

HEALTH EXPENDITURE: Health expenditure in 2009 amounted to EUR 15.7 billion. The public sector is the main source of health funding, 74.7% of health spending was funded by public sources in 2009 slightly more than the average of 71.7% in OECD countries. The share of public spending in Finland was however lower than in all other Nordic countries where it exceeds 80%. As in other OECD countries the health expenditure has been growing steadily since the year 2000. In 2009 health spending per capita in Finland is equal to the OECD average with spending of EUR 2936. Municipalities spent on average about 1300 Euros per inhabitant on health care in 2005. Health care accounted for about 25% of the municipal budget. In a comparison of 16 countries in 2008 Finland used the least resources and attained average results, making Finland the most efficient public sector health service producer. One of the possible explanations for the low total health care expenditures in Finland is the low salary of health care professionals, especially the nurses.

PRIVATE SECTOR: Due to the comprehensive public sector, private health care sector is relatively small. Between 3-4% of in-patient care is provided by the private health care system. Physiotherapy, dentistry, and occupational health services are the most often used health services in the private sector. Approximately 105 of medical doctors work solely in the private sector Although higher user fees may cause a barrier to using private sector services as most is paid out-of-pocket, a significant share of the cost is reimbursed by the Social Insurance Institution. Employers are obliged by law to provide occupational health care services for their employees as are educational establishments for their students and staff.

NATIONAL HEALTH INSURANCE: The statutory National Health Insurance (NHI) scheme covers all Finnish residents and it is run by the Social Insurance Institution(SII) through approximately about 260 local offices all over the country. The responsibilities of this institute include coverage of some family benefits, National Health Insurance, rehabilitation basic unemployment security, housing benefits, financial aid for students and state guaranteed pensions. The NHI system offers varying levels of reimbursement for out patient drugs, care from private providers, transport costs to health care facilities, sickness and maternity leave allowances, and some rehabilitation services. The NHI also partially reimburses occupational healthcare costs for services delivered to employees but not to dependents.

Additional voluntary health insurance has a very marginal role in the Finnish health care system and is mainly used to supplement the reimbursement rate of NHI,

PHARMACEUTICALS: Out-patient pharmaceuticals, including over-the-counter drugs can only be sold to patients by pharmacies. Providers can only deliver drugs that are actually administered within their facilities. Health centers can give outpatient drugs when local pharmacies are closed but only in the dosage needed to cover the time until the pharmacy reopens. Finland limits medicine sales to about 800 licensed pharmacies. Electronic prescribing is used in about half the pharmacies but all are expected to have the capability during 2012.

HEALTH INFORMATION TECHNOLOGY: Electronic Patient Records (EPR) have been in use since 2007 virtually in every heath care provider, however it is not coordinated nationally partly due to a decentralized health care system. Efforts are underway to create a common, national structure for communication between patients and providers over the internet. The Finnish Office for health Technology Assessment is an independent public assessment agency working as part of the National Institute of Health and Welfare since 1995. The aim is to assist decision-making by supplying information that is of a high scientific standard. The service is for all professional groups in health care, political decision-makers and the general public and to provide an appraisal of foreign results in local conditions. Immigrants who live in Finland permanently are also entitled to the same services as the Finnish people.

ORGANIZATIONAL STRUCTURE: Health care policy is primarily the field of Ministry of Social Affairs and Health. Due to decentralized public administration, municipalities decide themselves how the local services are provided. Every municipality has a responsibility to offer health services to their residents and it is usually provided at municipal health care centers. Primary care is obtained from the health care centers employing general practitioners and nurses who provide most day-to-day medical services. The general practitioners are also the gatekeepers to the more specialized services in the secondary and tertiary care centers. Secondary care is provided by the municipalities through district hospitals. Finland has a network of five university teaching hospitals which make up the tertiary level. These contain the most advanced medical equipment and facilities in the country. These are funded by the community but national government meets the cost of medical training.

The private sector provides one third of the specialized out patient services and around 8% of the inpatient services. Patients pay most of the cost of private health services while part of the fee may be reimbursed by the compulsory Sickness Insurance Scheme.

HEALTH CARE IN THE REPUBLIC OF IRELAND

The public health care system of Ireland is governed by the Health Act of 2004 which established a new body to be responsible for health and personal social services to everyone living in Ireland—the Health Service Executive. The new national health service came into being officially on 1 Jan, 2005: however the new structures are currently in the process of being established as the reform program continues. In addition to the public sector there is also a large private sector.

In 2005 Ireland spent 8.2%of GDP on health care or US $ 3,996 per capita. Of that approximately 79% was government expenditure.

HEALTH CARE SYSTEM: All persons resident in Ireland are entitled to receive health care through the public health care system which is managed by the Health Service Executive and funded by general taxation. A person may be required to pay a subsidized fee for certain health care received; this depends on income, age, illness or disability. All maternity services and child care up to the age of six months are provided free of charge. Emergency care is provided at a cost of 100 Euros for a visit to the Accident and Emergency department. Everyone living in the country, and visitors to Ireland who hold a European Health Insurance Card, are entitled to free maintenance and treatment in public beds in Health Service Executive and voluntary hospitals. Out patient services are also provided for free. However the majority of patients on median incomes and above are required to pay subsidized hospital charges.

The *Medical Card:* which entitles holder to free hospital care, GP visits, dental services, optical services aural services, prescription drugs, and medical appliances is available to those receiving welfare payments, low earners, those with certain long-term or severe illnesses and in certain other cases. Many political parties support extending the availability of the medical card to eventually cover everyone resident in Ireland—they currently cover 31.9%. of the population. Those on slightly higher incomes are eligible for the GP Visit Card which entitles the holder to free general practitioner visits. For persons over 70 years who are not entitled to a medical card or GP visit card they instead receive an annual cash grant of 400 Euros up to a certain income. People who are not entitled to a Medical Card (68%of the population) must pay fees for certain health services. There is 100 Euros A&E charge for those who attend an accident and emergency department without a referral letter from a family doctor (a visit to which usually costs 50-75 Euros.) Hospital charges (for inpatients) are a flat fee of 100Euros per day up to a maximum of 1000 Euros in any twelve month period, irrespective of the actual care received. Specialist assessments and diagnostic assessments (such as x-rays, laboratory tests physiotherapy, etc) are provided for free. If a person cannot afford to pay hospital charges, the HSE will provide the services free of charge.

HOSPITALS: Many hospitals in Ireland are operated directly by the HSE. There are hospitals run on a voluntary basis by organizations. Some are teaching hospitals (such as University College Hospital, Galway) operated in conjunction with a university. There are also many private hospitals. Hospitals in Ireland generally offer a full range of health care including accident and emergency services.

WAITING LISTS: The public health system, despite massive expenditures in recent years, has some problems. An ongoing issue is the "waiting lists" for those requiring, in some cases, serious operations. In 2007 76% of inpatients were admitted to hospital immediately, 11% had to wait up to one month, 4% had to wait up to three months, 1% had to wait up to six months and 4% had to wait over six months for operations. For outpatients 23% were seen on time, 44% were seen within 30 minutes, 18% waited more than an hour and 7% waited two hours.

The National Treatment Purchase Fund was set up in 2002 for those waiting over 3 months for an operation or procedure and as a result over 135,000 patients on waiting lists have been treated so far. The NTPF involves the government paying for public patients to be treated for free in a private hospital in Ireland, or sometimes abroad if necessary. The NTPF has reduced waiting times for procedures to an average of between two to five months (with the average in 2009 being 2.4 months) compared to between two and five years in 2002.

HEALTH CENTERS: Health centers provide a wide range of primary care and community services in towns and villages throughout Ireland, and are run by HSE. Services available at these clinics include GP services, public health nurses, social services, child protection services, child health services, community welfare, disability services, older people services, chiropody, ophthalmic, speech therapy, addiction counseling and treatment, physiotherapy, occupational therapy, psychiatric services, Home Help and more. These services are available for free or at a subsidized rate.

GENERAL PRACTITIONERS: Primary care in Ireland is mostly provided by general practitioners (GPs) who generally operate as solo traders or in health centers with other GPs and sometimes nurses. Most GPs also offer house visits to their patients, with there being "emergency" out-of-hours GP services available in all parts of the country. GPs generally charge on a per consultation fee basis usually charging anything up to 60 euros. People with Medical Cards or GP Visit Cards are exempt from charges. Many GPs also provide services to those with Hepatitis C and maternity and infant services for free. Those with private health insurance can, depending on their plan, get their GP costs paid for or refunded either fully or partially by the insurance company. People can also claim tax relief for GP costs.

DRUGS: Prescription drugs and medical appliances are available to all for free or at a reduced cost. The 'Drugs Payment Scheme' ensures that every household only has to pay, maximum, 120 Euros per calendar month for up to a maximum of one month's supply of prescribed drugs, medicines and medical appliances. Those who hold medical cards, suffering from long-term illnesses or who have hepatitis C do not have to pay any thing for medicines or appliances. All immunization vaccines for children are provided free of charge and are provided in schools, health clinics or hospitals. Recovering heroin addicts are able to get methadone treatment for free under the 'Methadone Treatment Scheme'

OTHER SERVICES: The HSE provide dental, optical (vision) and aural (hearing) health care. Medical Card holders and their dependents, 'Health Amendment Act' Card holders and children get these services free. Other people can get these services free or at a reduced cost from the 'Treatment Benefit Scheme' and/or private insurance, or claim tax relief after paying the full cost with a private practitioner. The HSE also provide mental health services and treatment and rehabilitation services for alcohol and drug addicts.

PAYMENT SCHEMES: Those without a Medical Card or private health insurance are able to receive medical services for free or at a subsidized rate from the 'Treatment Benefit Scheme'—as are their dependents which brings into account the compulsory 'Social Insurance Fund' (PRSI) contributions they have made. People can also claim tax relief on medical expenses that are not covered by the state or by private health insurance. Those with private health insurance also get tax credits, which are passed directly on to the insurance company and lower the customer's premium. Visitors to Ireland who hold a European Health Card do not have to pay anything for emergency treatment from a general practitioner or specialist, emergency dental, oral or aural treatment, inpatient or outpatient hospital treatment or prescription medicines. Those who need dialysis, oxygen therapy or other such treatments can arrange for it before their visit.

SATISFACTION WITH THE HEALTH SERVICE: A survey, commissioned by the HSE in 2007, found that patient satisfaction with the health service was quite high with 90% of inpatients and 85% of outpatients saying they were satisfied with their treatment. In addition to this, 97 % said they were satisfied with the care provided by their GP.

The 2008 Health Consumer Powerhouse *EURO HEALTH CONSUMER INDEX* report ranked Ireland's public healthcare system 11th out of 31 European countries. This is an improvement over the 2006 report, in which Ireland was ranked 26th out of 26 countries.

HEALTH SERVICE EXECUTIVE: The Health Service Executive (HSE) manages the delivery of the entire health service as a single national entity. There are four HSE administrative areas which in turn are divided into 32 local health offices. The HSE is Ireland's largest employer with over 100,000 workers and has an annual budget 0f 16 billion Euros, more than any other public sector organization.

MINISTER FOR HEALTH AND CHILDREN: The minister for health and children has responsibility for setting overall policy with regard to the health service.

PRIVATE HEALTH INSURANCE: Private health insurance is available to the population for those who want it. In 2005, 47.6% of people were covered by private health insurance. The regulatory body for private health insurance is the Health Insurance Authority. The Hospital Saturday Fund is also available to give customers cash towards a range of every day health care costs.

HEALTH STATISTICS: * 47.6 % of Ireland's population were covered by private health insurance and 31.9% were covered by Medical Cards. * 23% of the population over 16 had a chronic illness or health problem. 19.6 % of the population over 16 had limited activity. *47.2% of the population over 16 described their health as *'very good'* *35.7% as "good". *24.9% of the population over 16 were classed as smokers. *There were 53 publicly funded acute hospitals, with a total of 12,094 in-patient beds available, 1,253 day beds available, and the average length of an in-patient stay in hospital was 6.6 days.

HEALTHCARE IN ALGERIA

Health in Algeria, according to information from a march 6, 2006 United States report, does not compare well with the developed world. Algeria has inadequate numbers of physicians (one per 1000 people) and hospital beds (2.1 per 1000people) and poor access to water (87% of the population) and sanitation (92% of the population). Given Algeria's young population, policy favors preventive health care and clinics over hospitals. In keeping with this policy the government maintains an immunization program. However poor sanitation and unclean water still cause tuberculosis, hepatitis, measles, typhoid fever, cholera and dysentery. In 2003 about 0.10 % of the population aged 15-49 was living with human immunodeficiency virus / acquired immune deficiency syndrome (HIV/AIDS). The poor generally receive health care free of charge, but the wealthy pay for care according to a sliding scale. Access to health care is enhanced by the requirement that doctors and dentists work in public health for at least five years. However doctors are more easily found in the cities of the north than in the southern Sahara region.

The Ministry of health has overall responsibility for the health sector, although the Ministry of Defense runs some military hospitals. In 1990 Algeria had 284 hospitals with 60,124 beds (2.4 per1000 people, as of 1999 this ratio had declined to an estimate of 2.1) there were also 1309 health centers, 510 polyclinics, and 475 maternity hospitals (64 privately owned) in 1990. Medical personnel included 23,550 doctors, 2134 pharmacists, and 7,199 dentists. As of 1999 there was an estimated 1 physician per 1,000 people and total health care expenditure was estimated at 3.6% of GDP.

Free medical care was introduced in 1974 under a social security system that reimburses 80% of private consultation and prescription drugs. The principal health problems have been tuberculosis, malaria, trachoma, and malnutrition. By 1999 the incidence of tuberculosis was 45 in 100,000. In 2000, the average life expectancy was 71 years with a death rate of 5.2 per 1000 people. Infant mortality in 2000 was 33 per 1000 live births and estimated maternal mortality as of 1998 was220 per 100,000 live births. The government is interested in creating public awareness of birth control. As of 2000 an estimated 51% of women ages 15 to 49 were using some form of contraception. The total fertility rate decreased to 3.2 in 2000 from 5.0 in 1987. Malnutrition was present in an estimated 18% of all children under the age of five according to figures available as of 2000. The HIV prevalence among adults in 2000 was only 0.7 per 100 adults. As of 1995 only 214 cases were reported. Algeria's immunization rates as of 1999 for one year old children were: diphtheria, pertussis, and tetanus, 83% and measles 83%,. In 2000 94% of the population had access to adequate sanitation.

HEALTH IN MOROCCO

According to the United States government, Morocco has an inadequate number of men physicians 0.5 per 1000 people and hospital beds (1per 1000 people), and poor access to water (82% of the population).and sanitation (75% of the population). The health care system includes 122 hospitals, 2,400 health centers, and 4 university clincs, but they are poorly maintained and lack adequate capacity to meet the demand for medical care. Only 24,000 beds are available for 6 million people seeking care each year, including 3 million emergency cases. The health budget corresponds to 1.1 percent of gross domestic product and 5.5% of the central government budget.

MATERNAL AND CHILD HEALTH CARE: In June 2011the United Nations Population Fund released a report on the state of the world's Midwifery. The 2010 maternal mortality rate per 100,000 births for Moroccoins 110. This is compared with 124 in 2008, and 383 in 1990. The under 5 mortality per 1000 births is 39 and the neonatal mortality as a percentage of under 5's mortality is 54. In Morocco the number of midwives per 1000 live births is 5 and 1 in 360 is the lifetime risk of death for pregnant women.

DISEASE: In 2001 the principal causes of mortality in the urban population were circulatory system diseases (20%) perinatal diseases (9.3%).; cancer (8.5%); endocrinological, nutritional, and metabolic diseases (7.6%); respiratory system diseases (6.9%); and infectious and parasitic diseases (4.7%). In 2004 the ministry of health announced that the country had eradicated a variety of childhood diseases, specifically diphtheria, polio, tetanus, and malaria, but other diseases pose challenges. Although still high at more than 40 deaths per 1000 live births in 2006 the infant mortality rate shows considerable improvement since 1981 when it was estimated at 91 deaths per 1000 live births. According to estimates for 2001 approximately 0.1 percent of the population between the ages of 15 and 49 was infected with human immunodeficiency virus/ acquired immune deficiency syndrome (HIV/AIDS)

According to the last census, Morocco has a population approaching 30 million. 55% of the population is living in urban areas. The Moroccan population is young with 38% under the age of 14 years, and life expectancy at birth has increased from 65 to 68.5 in2004. The country has made good progress in the control of preventable childhood disease but social and health inequalities remain major problems. The country still ranks 125th according to the human development index(HDI)(UNDP 2004). This position is explained by low income, high adult illiteracy, lack of generalized education, and health indicators. There is difficult access to basic social services such as education and health.

The Moroccan system of health care is organized into three sectors

* The public health care sector. This the largest sector present throughout the country, providing 85% of the country's hospital beds and representing the main employer of health professionals in the country. This sector is supposed to deal with the needs of the poor and rural population who are unable to afford the service offered by the private sector.
* The private health care sector. This is a profit-making sector which is mainly present in the cities. It is principally attended by people with sufficient income or those who have insurance.
* The non-profit health sector. This sector is present exclusively in the cities and run mainly by the National Security Fund (CNSS) Its care is devoted to the 16%of the population covered by health insurance.

During the past four decades the budget devoted to health represented on average 1% of GDP each year and bad governance of an ill health system. Only 40% of births are attended by skilled personnel. Many women continue to die during childbirth and infant mortality rate remains high. With an average of one doctor for 2100 inhabitants Morocco compares badly with countries of equivalent level of development. Inequities are found between cities and rural areas. The number of doctors can vary between one doctor for 840 inhabitants to one doctor for 4600 in another region. The global health expenditure is very low and mainly supported by households(60%) whereas 40% of all expenditure engaged by the health ministry goes to the richest 20% of the population. Health insurance covers only 16% of the population nearly exclusively in the cities. This percentage is expected to increase to 32% under the new law on Compulsory Health Insurance supposed to be applicable by 2006. In 1999 the percentage of the population with sustainable access to affordable essential drugs was estimated to be between 50 % and 79 %. More than 33% are unable to afford medical care. The inequity is exacerbated in rural areas where the percentage reaches 44%. Inequities also exist for the free access to public structures since the richest are more likely to get free care than the poorest. Households devote an average 6.5% of their budget to health care. This becomes 9% for the poorest 20% whereas it represents 3.9% for the richest 20%. Health care is becoming less and less affordable. The cost for an insulin dependent diabetic is estimated at 120 dollars per month. This is nearly the monthly wages of a non-qualified manual laborer. According to one study the prevalence of hypertension, hypercholesterolemia and diabetes were respectively 33.6%, 29%, and 6.6 %. The prevalence of obesity was markedly higher in females in urban areas with 40% of women overweight. Sexually transmitted disease, and environmental related diseases such as tuberculosis, typhoid, viral hepatitis, trachoma, and conjunctivitis have been persistent or increasing during the last six years.

HEALTH CARE IN IRAN

The cost of health care in Iran was almost US $ 24 Billion in 2002 and was forecast to rise to US $ 31 billion by 2007. With a population of almost 70 million, Iran is one of the most populous countries in the Middle East. This country faces the common problem of other young demographic nations in the region which is keeping pace with growth of an already huge demand for various public services. The young population will soon be old enough to start new families, which will boost the population growth rate and subsequently the need for public health infrastructure and services. Total healthcare spending is expected to rise from 24.3 billion in 2008 to 50 billion by 2013 reflecting the increasing demand on medical services. Total health spending was equivalent to 4.2% of GDP in Iran in2005, 73 % of all Iranians have healthcare coverage.

The World Health Organization in the last report on health systems ranks Iran's performance on health level, and it's overall health system performance 93rd among the world's nations. The status of Iranians has improved over the last two decades. Iran has been able to extend public health preventive services through the establishment of an extensive Primary Health Care Network. As a result child and maternal mortality rates have fallen significantly, and life expectancy at birth has risen remarkably. Infant and under five mortality have decreased to 28.6 and 35.6 per 1000 live births respectively in 2000, compared to an Infant mortality of 122 per 1000 and an under 5 mortality of 191 per 1000 in 1970. Immunization of children is accessible to most of the urban and rural population. Life expectancy in 2010 was 71.4 years

Coverage: The constitution entitles Iranians to basic health care and most receive subsidized prescription drugs and vaccination programs. An extensive network of public clinics offers basic care at low cost, and general and specialty hospitals operated by the ministry of health and education provide higher levels of care. In most large cities, well-to-do persons use private clinics, and hospitals that charge high fees. About 73% of all Iranians workers have health care and social security coverage. Between 80% and 94% of the population could access affordable essential medicines in 1999. Since 2009, a new government plan called the "comprehensive insurance plan" provides basic coverage to all Iranians. Iran has been very successful in training /educating the necessary human resources for its health system. The system of almost 30 years ago when the country was facing a shortage of all kinds of skilled personnel in the health and medical sector has been completely changed into one in which the necessary professionals now completely suffice the country's needs. There are now 488 government funded hospitals in Iran. There are now 51 Medical Schools; 1 million medical students; 120,000 hospital beds; 100,000 doctors; 170,000 nurses, 20,000 village clinics; and 20,000 professors of medicine.

HEALTH NETWORK IN IRAN: Today the largest healthcare network is owned and run by the Ministry of Health and Medical Education(MOHME) through its network of health establishments and medical schools in the country. MOHME is in charge of provision of healthcare services through its network: Medical insurance, medical education, supervision and regulation of the healthcare system in the country, policymaking, production and distribution of pharmaceuticals, and research and development. Additionally, there are other parallel organizations such as Medical Services Insurance Organizations (MSIO) that have been established to act as a relief foundation as well as an insurance firm. Some hospitals, such as Mahak for children's cancer are run by charitable foundations. According to the last census in 2003 Iran possesses 730 medical establishments with a total of 111,000 beds of which 77,300 beds are directly affiliated and run by MOHME and 11,300 owned by the private sector and the rest belong to other organizations such as the Social Security Organization of Iran(SSO). There are about seven nurses and 17 hospital beds per 10,000 population. An elaborate system of health network has been established which has ensured provision of primary health care to the vast majority of the public though access is somewhat limited in the lesser developed provinces.

DEVELOPMENT: Although overall improvements have been achieved in all health areas since the 1979 revolution, the present challenging economic conditions of the country combined with rapid advances in medical technology and information technology, Individuals' expectations and the young demographic of the population will challenge the sustainability of the improvements thus far. Iran is the 19th country in medical research (2012).

Iran has a medical tourism attraction and 30,000 people come to Iran each year to receive medical treatment

WATER AND SANITATION: Iran has one of the highest percentages of population in the Middle East with access to safe drinking water, with an estimated 92% of its people enjoying such access (Nearly 100% in urban areas and about 80% in rural areas) as of 2007. There is a considerable shortfall in wastewater treatment; for example in Tehran the majority of the population has no wastewater treatment, with raw sewage being injected directly into groundwater. With an expanding population, the pollution of groundwater causes increasing health risks.

NUTRITION: Despite the fact that Iran consists of an agrarian economy, there is a high degree of malnutrition within the country. Approximately one fourth of all young children have stunted or wasted growth characteristics due to undernourishment, moreover as an indicator of the poor food distribution capability the percentage of undernourished children in villages is much higher. About 13% of young people are classified as obese according to United Nations FAO sources. According to the government of Iran about 60% of Iranians are overweight and 35% of women and 15% of men are obese. The soft drinks industry is valued at 2 billion dollars a year and consumption at 46 liters per capita.

COMMUNICABLE DISEASES & DRUGS: Cholera has been a persistent problem in Iran. The 2005 epidemic involved the loss of many lives and television warned people not to eat vegetables. The 1998 epidemic involved considerably more cases and loss of life. Increased drug use has driven up the incidence of immunodeficiency virus infection (HIV). In 2005 two-thirds of the official total were attributed to drug use. Iran has an HIV treatment system. According to the United Nations Aids in Iran has been increasing at a rapid rate. Drug use has been the major factor however. There is an increase in sexual transmission of the disease. In 2009 men account for 93% of the HIV patients and women comprise 7% of the infected population. The rate of the infection is still very low compared to international standards. Iran has a rate of about 0.16 % of the adult population (18000 cases) compared with 0.8 per cent in North America (2008). But according to the WHO as of 2009 there are more than 100,000 aids sufferers in Iran.

DRUG ADDICTION: Drug addiction constitutes a major health problem. Iran is situated along one of the main trafficking routes for cannabis, heroin, opium, and morphine produced in Afghanistan. Designer drugs have also found their way into the local market in recent years. Iran ranks first worldwide in the prevalence of opiate addiction with 2.8% of its population addicted. Initiation age for most Iranian addicts is in their 20s. Of the 7,700 tons of opium produced in Afghanistan 3000 tons entered Iran. Iran discovers 3 tons of drugs daily. In 2005 estimates of the number of drug addicts ranged from 2to 4 million. Reasons for addiction include lack of economic prospects and lack of freedom. The drug problem inflicts an annual damage of about 8.5 billion dollars on Iran's economy.

SMOKING: About 20% of adult male and 4.5% of adult female population in the country smoke tobacco (12,000,000 smokers) Smoking is responsible for 25% of the deaths in the country), 60,000 Iranians die directly or indirectly due to smoking every year (2008). Iranians spend more than 1.8 billion a year on tobacco. Smoking bans are currently in force for all public places, for drivers, for the traditional Persian waterpipe, and selling tobacco to anyone under 18 years of age.

AIR POLLUTION: The prevalence of respiratory disease and cancers in Iran is increasing at a significant rate, also because of air pollution in Tehran. The World Bank estimates losses inflicted on Iran's economy as a result of deaths caused by air pollution at $640 million.

LEADING CAUSES OF MORTALITY: According to Ministry of Health and Medical Education the leading causes of death in 2003 were due to diseases of the circulatory system(41%) and cancer. Myocardial infarction was the cause of 25% of deaths. Addiction is the fourth major cause of death in Iran following road accidents, heart disease, and depression.

PHARMACEUTICALS: The pharmaceutical industry in Iran began in its modern form in 1920, when the Pasteur Institute was founded. Iran has a well developed pharmaceutical production capability though it still relies on imports for raw materials and many specialized drugs. Iran's Ministry of Health and Medical Education(MOHE) has a mission to provide access to sufficient quantities of safe, effective and high quality medicines that are affordable for the entire population. Since the 1979 revolution Iran has adopted a full generic-based National drug policy, with local production of essential drugs and vaccines. Although over 85% of the population uses an insurance system to reimburse their drug expenses the government heavily subsidizes pharmaceutical production / importation in order to increase affordability of medicines, which tends also to increase overconsumption, over-prescription and misuse of drugs, such as antibiotics. The MOHME is the main stakeholder of pharmaceutical affairs in the country. Iran has produced a wide range of pharmaceuticals for the treatment of cancer, diabetes, infection and depression. In recent years several drugmakers have developed the ability to innovate away from generic drug production itself.

MEDICAL EQUIPMENT: The department of Medical Equipments in the Ministry of Health and Medical Education (MOHMR) is responsible for supervising imports of medical equipment but the distribution of such equipment is handled by the private sector. Iran has undergone the primary stages of industrialization and a strong indigenous manufacturing capability now exists in the country. One can expect to find a handful of local producers for basic medical equipment. 'Iran MED' 'and Iran LAB' are the main annual exhibitions relating to medical and laboratory equipments in Tehran. In 2009

$3.1 billion worth of drugs and medical products were consumed in Tehran. In 2009, Iran exported $74 million worth of "medical products" to countries such as Iraq, Afganistan, and Russia. There are over 100 Iranian companies representing the international suppliers in this market handling both promotion and after-sales service of the products. Iran is a mature market when it comes to medical equipment.

Healthcare in Switzerland

Health care in Switzerland is universal and is regulated by the Federal Health Insurance Act of 1994. Health insurance is compulsory for all persons residing in Switzerland (within 3 months of taking up residence or being born in the country) International civil servants and their family are exempted from compulsory health insurance. They can however, apply to join the Swiss health insurance system within 6 months of taking up residence in the country. Health insurance covers the cost of medical treatment and hospitalization of the insured. However the insured person pays part of the cost of treatment This is done (a) by means of an annual excess(or deductible called the 'franchise'). which ranges from CHF 300 to a maximum 2500 as chosen by the insured person (premiums are adjusted accordingly) and (b) by a charge of 10% of the costs over and above the excess up to a stop-loss amount of CHF 700.

Switzerland has an infant mortality rate of about 3.9 out of 1000. The general life expectancy for men is79.4 years compared with 84.2 for women.

COMPULSORY COVERAGE AND COSTS: Swiss are required to purchase basic health insurance, which covers a range of treatments detailed in the Federal Act. It is the same throughout the country and avoids double standards in healthcare. Insurers are required to offer this basic insurance to everyone, regardless of age or medical condition. They are not allowed to make a profit off this basic insurance, but can on supplemental plans. The insured pays the insurance premium for the basic plan up to 8% of their personal income. If a premium is higher than this, then the government gives the insured a cash subsidy to pay for any additional premium. The universal compulsory coverage provides for treatment in case of illness or accident (unless another accident insurance provides the cover) and pregnancy. Health insurance covers the costs of medical treatment and hospitalization of the insured. However, the insured person pays part of the cost of treatment. This is done

- By means of an annual excess(or deductible called the "franchise') which ranges from CHF 300 to a maximum of CHF 2500 as chosen by the insured person (premiums are adjusted accordingly);
- And by a charge of 10% of the costs over and above the excess. This is known as the retention, and is up to a maximum of 700CHF per year (excluding medication).

In case of pregnancy there is no charge. For hospitalization, one pays a contribution to room and service costs.

Insurance premiums vary from insurance company to company depending on the excess level chosen, the place of residence of the insured person, and the degree of supplementary coverage chosen(dental care private ward etc) In 2010, the average monthly compulsory basic health insurance premiums (with accident insurance).in Switzerland are:

* CHF 351.05 for an adult (age 26-years)
* CHF 293.85 for a young adult(age 19-25 years)
* CHF 84.03 for a child (age 0-18 years)

PRIVATE INSURANCE: The compulsory insurance can be supplemented by private "complementary" insurance policies that allow for coverage of some of the treatment categories not covered by the basic insurance or to improve the standard of room or service in case of hospitalization. This can include dental treatment and private ward hospitalization which are not covered by the compulsory insurance. As far as the compulsory health insurance is concerned, the insurance companies cannot set any conditions relating to age, sex, or state of health for coverage. Although the level of premium can vary from one company to another they must be identical within the same company for all insured persons of the same age group and region, regardless of sex or state of health. This does not apply to complementary insurance, where premiums are risk-based.

ORGANIZATION: The Swiss healthcare system is a combination of public, subsidized private, and totally private systems:

- Public: e.g. the University of Geneva Hospital with 2350 beds, 8300 staff and 50,000 patients a year:
- Subsidized private: the home care services to which one may have recourse in case of a difficult pregnancy or childbirth, illness, handicap or old age;
- Totally private: doctors in private practice and in private clinics.

The insured person has full freedom of choice among the recognized healthcare providers competent to treat their condition, on the understanding that the costs are covered by the insurance up to the level of the official tariff. There is freedom of choice when selecting an insurance company (provided that it is registered and authorized by the Federal Act.) to which one pays a premium, usually on a monthly basis.

STATISTICS: Healthcare Costs in Switzerland are 10.8 % of GDP; out-of-pocket healthcare payments average US$1,350.

Comments

This review while hardly exhaustive does direct our attention to what works, what works best, and in many cases what does not work well and needs change. There is little doubt that every country or society with a government or ruling class needs to organize and provide for the health care of its population. In fact all the national designs for healthcare differ. Most differ from each other significantly in the way the plan is organized, how much the government is responsible for, how much is private, how much is covered by insurance, how much of the cost is born by the patient, the government, the insurance or the special program for a special part of the population e. g. Medicare and Social Security in the USA; special groups of patients such as renal failure and dialysis or maternity or accidents. Some have a cap on how much a person has to pay according to age and income. Others require or would like to require employers to carry part of the burden as a benefit of employment. It does not seem to be easy to devise a simple system that covers everyone since everyone needs the same level of care and the same access to medical care and the degree of expertise for the problem whether it be in a clinic, in a private room or ward, without those nagging and irritable delays for diagnostic radiology and necessary surgery. Then there is the burden of cost to achieve these noble and necessary objectives. The USA some how requires twice as much per capita expenditure as the rest of the world. Cost is an annual and perennial problem and the cause of much debate for the legislature or Ministry about what is affordable and what is necessary. Then there are the technological innovations that may change how doctors and their assistants monitor patients and guide their activities. We now have online groups for support and advice. There is a growing community of "quantified selfers" who monitor their own bodily functions and discuss their results. This is viewed as a possible cost control item. Needless to say that cost control seems to be paramount in all national systems. Delays in treatment or surgery are an ever-present problem in socialized systems such as in Canada. This may lead to some medical or surgical tourism as from Canada to the United States. Some medical tourism occurs because of cost as well as delays e. g. heart surgery in India. To some extent medicine is practiced over the telephone, the mobile phone, the internet, and television. These are still extremes and not likely to replace talking to and being examined by a health professional in the office, clinic or hospital. One current example of medical tourism is medical care sought in Mexico by nearly 1 million Californians annually. Another example of high health care costs at home driving Californians to seek medical care in a foreign country. They seek medical, dental and prescription services. Many of these are Mexican immigrants but some are US citizens all of whom don't have health insurance. This information is based on 2001 study by the California Health Interview Survey.

How the doctors survive and practice in this atmosphere of severe austerity, malpractice suites, Medicare threats and lowered fees, reimbursement reductions by insurance companies, and the high overhead of private office practice, patients who don't or cannot pay as well as the stress of all these financial threats to say nothing of just the professional burdens is yet to be seen. There seems to be a growing tendency to leave private solo practice for practice as employees of hospitals (hospitalists), large groups, corporations, and the government such as state, federal, VA, Tricare, even the military. As a friend once described her experience in private practice—"the first 10 years I made money; the second 10 years I lost money and now I work for the government". A salaried job without the rent, salaries, malpractice insurance costs and the need to run a corporate entity in addition to the many professional requirements is appealing and sometimes life-saving. There is little question for instance that Medicare, Medicaid, and the Insurance companies pay better though not full value for procedures than they do for office visits, time spent with a patient, or consultations. This puts the Family Practitioner or the Internist at a disadvantage.

An interesting commentary on why medical care in the US is so much more expensive (2x more than other industrialized nations) than the rest of the world was published by a vascular surgeon (Frank Veith MD) and a cardiologist (Zvonimir Krajcer MD) in a Surgery News 2010 publication. These are experienced and prominent members of the academic community. Some of their comments may be hard to believe and do not offer a complete picture of medical economics but are certainly part of the picture: 1. Building Shrines for hospital administrators. Both witnessed the building of expensive new healthcare facilities for which they felt there was no real need, to satisfy an institutional desire to provide a monument to a hospital executive. In one case, a billion dollar architecturally spectacular new hospital buildings were erected within a few hundred yards of similar facilities belonging to a competing institution. In another case a specialty hospital was constructed when two similar specialty facilities belonging to a competing institution existed within a few miles. In both instances the costs of the buildings were large but relatively minor compared with the cost the duplicate staffing required for these unnecessary and marginally used new facilities. Moreover, to keep both new facilities acceptably occupied, substantial additional monies continue to be spent on advertising and public relations. 2: Unnecessary duplication of services. A large city had three excellent transplant programs. A fourth university hospital also wanted a transplant program to enhance its reputation and prestige. When the relevant state agency determined that there was no need for a fourth transplant program in the city, the medical center's president interceded with a high ranking elected state official with whom he had a political relationship. As a result the unneeded fourth program was quickly approved. The costs for the complex and extensive additional staffing and equipment for the extra program were borne by our healthcare system. Since the number of organ transplants in the area is totally dependent on the number of donor organs and not on the number of programs, no increase in quality or number of patients treated could accrue. The sole purpose served by the additional program was gratification of institutional ego needs. 3: Absence of medical malpractice tort reform. It is well known that medical liability costs are out of control in New York State. Abuses are rampant since the system depends on contingency payments to trial lawyers and "hired gun" expert witnesses who are often non-expert and are paid handsomely for their biased opinions, a pure example of conflict of interest. Numerous studies have documented that most awards, some larger than lottery payouts, do not correlate at all with actual malpractice and most instances of actual malpractice do result in awards. Clearly the system is fueled by greedy lawyers who contribute large sums of money to the campaigns of federal and state officials so that they will block reform of a system that is non-functional and exceedingly expensive. The insurance premium burden is passed on to the cost of our health care system. Worse still there are the staggering costs of defensive medical practices such as adding otherwise unnecessary tests, hospitalizations, and consultations. These defensive practices are estimated to increase health care costs by $65 billion to $200 billion a year. California and Texas have passed sensible state malpractice reform laws that protect patients' rights to seek redress for real malpractice while limiting liability to reasonable amounts rather than lottery amounts. President Bush and president Obama have both backed away from federal medical liability reform legislation. This problem needs to be addressed if we are serious about cutting health care costs.

Another item in the discussion by Veith and Krajcer is the reality that hospitals need to be in the black. Hospitals need to survive and cannot operate at a deficit. In order to avoid this they must admit enough insured and paying patients to maintain their income stream. Tremendous pressure is therefore placed on physicians and surgeons to increase hospital admissions. In one New York institution, salaried staff surgeons were ordered to increase their admissions and operations by 22% or face a cut in salary. Since most surgeons normally operate on patients who have appropriate indications for aggressive treatment the only way these surgeons could possibly increase their operative load is to perform operations that are not indicated or necessary. This subjects patients to unneeded risks and increases medical cost.

Decreased physician reimbursement: Decreased physician reimbursement leads to unnecessary procedures. Physicians like other human beings resist pay cuts. Physicians who do procedures are paid on the number of procedures performed. If the compensation per procedure is decreased—as is happening—the only way for a physician to maintain his or her income is to do more procedures. Accordingly a cut in procedural reimbursement will inevitably motivate physicians to do more procedures. This will result in an increase in unnecessary operations, increased costs and unnecessary risks to patients will result.

Pay for Performance: To improve the Quality of health care and physician performance, financial incentives have been proposed. These provide additional income to physicians who can perform procedures with lower mortality and morbidity rates. It is well known that patients who really need certain procedures are at higher risk of death and complications than are patients whose indications are weaker or nonexistent. Physicians therefore have an incentive to add easier cases regardless of whether these patients even need the operation, so that their mortality and morbidity rates will be lower and they will receive higher reimbursement rates. This approach will add to the trend of treating patients unnecessarily and thereby increasing costs. It will also motivate physicians to deny interventional or operative treatment to patients who really need it.

These are the experience, observations and interpretations of real life events and experience of two highly qualified physicians, one a famous vascular surgeon and one an academic experienced cardiologist. We need not agree with all their conclusions and interpretations as global truths but certainly their experience and conclusions about the state of affairs in medical economics and the medical practice must be taken seriously. Many situations play in the daily decisions that are made particularly in the realm of procedures. Many physicians and surgeons too accept the fact income is decreasing and cannot sustain private practice and either move to another job or retire. In other situations the surgeon may be pressed to take on cases that ordinarily might be rejected or referred elsewhere. One does not usually have control over the number of cases that present themselves. But these are only details in the overall cost picture.

By any measure, the United States spends an enormous amount of money on health care. Here are a few measures. In 2008 health care spending exceeded 16% of the nation's GDP. A comparison with other nations in 2004 reveals that the US spent 15.3% of GDP, while Canada spent 9.9%, France 10.7%, Germany 10.9% Sweden 9.1% and the United Kingdom 8.7%. The United States spent $6,037 per person, compared to Canada at $3,161, France at $3,191, Germany at $3,169, and the UK at $2,560. Those without health insurance face very high doctor and hospital bills with aggressive collection tactics. Those who are fortunate to have insurance are experiencing steep annual premium hikes along with rising deductibles and co-pays and all too often a well founded fear of losing their coverage should they lose their job or have a serious illness in the family. Americans may well underestimate the degree to which they subsidize the current US health care system out of their pocket. Almost no one knows that even people without health insurance pay substantial sums into the system today. If more people understood the full size of the health care bill that they are already paying for—and for a system that provides seriously inadequate care to millions of Americans—then the corporate opponents of a universal single-payer system might find it hard to frighten the public about the costs of that system. To recognize the advantages of a single-payer type system, we have to understand how the United States funds health care and health research and how much it actually costs. The US health care system is typically characterized as a largely private-sector system, so it may come as a surprise that more than 60% of the $2 trillion annual US health care bill is paid through taxes, according to a 2002 analysis published by Woolhandler and Himmelstein. Tax dollars pay for Medicare and Medicaid, for the Veterans Administration, the active and retired armed services and the Indian Health Service. Tax dollars pay for health coverage for federal, state, and municipal employees and their families, as well as for many employees of private companies working on government contracts. Less visible are the tax deductions for employer-paid health insurance along with other health-care related tax deductions, these also represent a form of government spending on health care. It makes little difference whether the government gives taxpayers (or their employers) a deduction for their Health care spending on the one hand, or collects their taxes then pays for their for their health care, either directly or via voucher on the other. Moreover tax dollars also pay for critical elements of the health care system apart from direct care—Medicare funds pay for much of the expensive equipment hospitals use, along with all medical residencies. All told, tax dollars already pay for at least $1.2 trillion in annual health care expenses. Since federal, state, and local governments collect $3.48 trillion dollars annually in taxes of all kinds—income, sales, property, corporate—that means that more than one third (34.4%) of the aggregate tax revenues collected in the United States go to pay for health care. Beyond their direct payments to health care providers and health insurance companies, Americans already make a sizeable annual payment into the health care system via taxes.

Facts and Figures Taken from the PNHP (Physicians for a National Health Program) Newsletter

> These figure and calculations are derived from an article by Joel Harrison for the PNHP SPRING NEWSLETTER 2009. Other calculations of the amount a household with an income of $25,000 going to health care (with insurance) for a family was $14,531(37%); If income level was $50,000 the cost to the family would be $17,406 (26.4%) on an annual basis. This does not include out of pocket expenses such as co-pays, deductibles and uncovered expenses. Some employers pay all of the premium others pay a percentage leaving much of the premium to the employee. These represent a significant bite out of the total wage packet. This becomes a bigger problem if insurance companies raise premiums, as they have recently following passage of *The Patient Protection and Affordable Care Act. (PPACA)*. In 2008 the US economy lost over 2 million jobs and 533,000 were lost in November alone. This was the biggest one month plunge in jobs in 34 years. This one month loss spells medical care disaster with millions of people losing their employer-sponsored health insurance joining the 46 million who did not have insurance coverage. *"PPACA"* is a mandate program that requires everyone to buy health insurance though not all can afford it. Meantime millions are finding it harder to pay their co-pays and deductibles and are scrimping on their medications and doctor visits. Many go without care. Experience with mandate-based-plans in

Washington state(1993), Oregon(1992), and Massachusetts (1998) shows that they simply don't work achieving neither universal health care nor cost containment. With private health insurance, universal coverage would be unaffordable. These companies generate immense overhead costs and force doctors and hospitals to spend heavily on billing and paperwork. Administration consumes about one third of every health care dollar in the US. By contrast in countries with non-profit national health insurance administrative costs consume only half that amount. Eliminating the private insurance industry would save $400 billion annually in administrative costs enough to ensure that everyone is covered and to eliminate all co-pays and deductibles. As we review the medical care plans of other nations we can see that several nations have achieved universal health care for all citizens and that usually includes visitors and migrants and are able to do this at about half the cost (percent of GDP or cost per capita). The US system does not cover all citizens (50 million uninsured) and still we pay twice as much as other industrialized countries. Are we getting more and better medical care? Are our doctors and other medical professionals so much better. The answer is no. But our insurance system unlike many other countries is a for profit system unlike Switzerland which has a no-profit insurance system. The US has a two trillion dollar system and rising. The insurance companies have calculated the increased costs of the Patient Protection And Affordable Care Act and have raised premiums in some cases like California as much as 25%. It is true that the new act specifies additional benefits and additional coverage such as limiting their ability to refuse coverage because of previous illness or disability, or prolonging coverage for children to age 26, or refusing to cover certain illnesses or hospitalization. We have not seen the end of premium increases because the new law does not become totally effective until 2015. The Affordable Care Act includes:

- 2010: Providing small business health insurance tax credits
- Allowing States to Cover More People on Medicaid
- Relief for Four Million Seniors Who Hit the Medicare Prescription Drug "Donut Hole"
- Cracking Down on Health Care Fraud
- Expanding Coverage for Early Retirees
- Providing Access to Insurance for uninsured Americans with Pre-Existing Conditions
- Putting Information for Consumers Online
- Extending Coverage for Young Adults
- Providing Free Preventive Care

- Prohibiting Insurance Companies from Rescinding Coverage
- Appealing Insurance Company Decisions
- Eliminating Lifetime Limits on Insurance Coverage
- Regulating Annual Limits on Insurance Coverage
- Prohibiting Denying Coverage of Children Based on Pre-existing Conditions
- Holding Insurance Companies Accountable for Unreasonable Rate Hikes
- Rebuilding the Primary Care Workforce
- Establishing Consumer Assistance Programs in the States
- Preventing Disease and Illness
- Strengthening Community Health Centers
- Payments for Rural Health Care Providers
- Prescription Drug Discounts
- 2011 Free Preventive Care for Seniors
- Bringing Down Health Care Premiums
- Addressing Overpayments to Big Insurance Companies and Strengthening Medicare Advantage
- Improving Health Care Quality and Efficiency
- Improving Care for Seniors After They Leave the Hospital
- New Innovations to Bring Down Costs
- Increasing access to Services at Home and in the Community
- Encouraging Integrated Health Systems
- 2012 Understanding and Fighting Health Disparities
- Providing New Voluntary Options for Long Term Care Insurance
- Reducing Paperwork and Administrative Costs
- Linking Payment to Quality Outcomes
- Improving Preventive Health Coverage
- 2013 Increasing Medicaid Payments for Primary Care Doctors
- Expanded Authority to Bundle Payments
- Additional Funding for the Children's Health Insurance Program (CHIP)
- Establishing Affordable Insurance Exchanges
- 2014 Promoting Individual Responsibility
- Ensuring Free Choice
- Increasing Access to Medicaid
- Makes Care More Affordable
- Ensuring Coverage for Individuals Participating In Clinical Trials
- Eliminating Annual Limits on Insurance Coverage

>   No Discrimination Due to Pre-Existing Conditions or Gender
>   Increasing Small Business Health Insurance Tax Credit
>   Paying Physicians Based on Value not Volume

2015

The above represent Goals and time table of the PATIENT PROTECTION AND AFFORDABLE CARE ACT. It is a mandated insurance plan basically run by for-profit insurance companies who will be free to adjust premiums to the needs of the company or corporation. It does not bode well for cost control.

Massachusetts passed a health care reform in 2006. The law was designed to extend coverage to virtually all state residents. Massachusetts' law mandates that uninsured individuals must purchase private insurance or pay a fine. The law established a new state agency to ensure that affordable plans were available; offered low income residents subsidies to help them buy coverage; and expanded Medicaid coverage for the very poor. (Immigrants are mostly excluded from the subsidies) Moneys that previously funded free care for the uninsured were shifted to the new insurance program, along with revenues from new fines on employers who fail to offer health benefits to their workers. In addition, the federal government provided extra funds for the programs first two years. Starting January 1, 2008 Massachusetts residents face fines if they cannot offer proof of insurance. Yet as of December 1,2007 only 37% of the 657,000 uninsured had gained coverage under the new program. These individuals often feel well served by the reform in that they now have insurance. However, 79% of the newly insured individuals are very poor people enrolled in Medicaid or similar free plans. Virtually all of them were previously eligible for completely free care funded by the state but face co-payments under the new plan. In effect, public funds for care of the poor that previously flowed directly to hospitals and clinics now flow through insurers with their higher administrative costs. Among the near poor uninsured (who are eligible for partial premium subsidies).only 16% had enrolled in the new coverage. And only 7% of the of the uninsured individuals with incomes too high to qualify for subsidies had enrolled according to official state figures. Few can afford premiums for even the skimpiest coverage; The lowest cost plan offered for a couple in their fifties costs $8200 annually, And carries a $2000 per person deductible.

The state's cost for subsidies is running $147 million over the $472 million budgeted for the fiscal year 2007. Meanwhile collections for fines on employers who fail to provide coverage are 80% below the original projections. The funding gap will probably widen in future years as the health care costs escalate and insurers raise premiums. State officials speak of raising co-pays and deductibles to make up the shortfall; and by slashing funds promised to safety net hospitals. While patients, the state, and safety net providers struggle, private insurers have prospered under the new law and the costs of bureaucracy have risen. Blue Cross the state's largest insurer is reaping more than a million dollars a day and awarded its chairman a $16.4 million retirement bonus even as he continues to draw a $3 million salary. All of the major insurers continue to charge overhead costs five times higher than Medicare and eleven-fold higher than Canada's single payer system. Moreover the new state agency that brokers private coverage adds its own surcharge of 4.5% to each policy it sells. A single payer program could save Massachusetts more than $9 billion annually on healthcare bureaucracy, making universal coverage affordable. Though this system is politically feasible, it is already proving fiscally unsustainable. The next economic downturn will increase the number of uninsured as tax revenues needed for the subsidies fall. The costs of the reform for the state have been formidable. Spending for the Commonwealth Care subsidized program has doubled from $630 million in 2007 to an estimated $1.3 Billion for 2009 which may not be sustainable. Reform of this design does not assure access to care because there is additional out-of-pocket expense in the form of co-payments that the patient or family cannot afford. Access to care is also affected by the uneven distribution of healthcare dollars between primary and specialty care hospitals. Agreements that tilt spending toward tertiary hospitals threaten the viability of community hospitals and health centers that provide a safety net for the uninsured and the underinsured. There is one US model of healthcare that meets the Institute of Medicine criteria for universal health care and that is Medicare.

INDIVIDUAL HEALTH BENEFIT ACCOUNTS

There are strong pressures for employers to pursue defined contribution health benefits with individual health benefit accounts such as Medical Savings Accounts (MSAs), Health Care Reimbursement Accounts (HCRAs) and Comprehensive Individual Medical Accounts (CIMAs). Health care consumers are becoming more assertive. The political backlash against managed care is eroding provider-based cost control mechanisms. Health insurance premium inflation is intensifying. Advocates of the movement toward individual health benefit accounts view them as a means of restoring autonomy to the physician-patient relationship and controlling costs. Opponents are concerned that individual health benefit accounts of any type will segment insurance markets, benefiting the healthy and wealthy at the expense of the chronically ill and the poor. A four year pilot federal legislation authorizing Medical Savings accounts (MSAs) expired.

MSA advocates say MSAs will

- Control costs without intrusion into the patient-physician relationship
- Reduce the number of uninsured by offering a low-cost, tax-exempt alternative to traditional health insurance
- Empower people with greater control over their health care and health—by allowing them to shop for high quality, low-cost care and by encouraging healthful lifestyles
- Improve satisfaction by offering wide choice of providers and scope of services
- Provide equal tax benefits to people who choose high out of-pocket insurance plans instead of low deductible plan

MSA opponents say:

- Mainly attract the healthy and wealthy-leaving the poor in traditional insurance with high premiums
- Attract people who are already insured, rather than the uninsured
- Provide a tax break for the wealthy that is so great it overshadows any positive health care effects
- Cause people to neglect preventive care

HEALTH CARE REIMBURSEMENT ACCOUNT

Healthcare Reimbursement Accounts (HCRAs) are not new. Despite this fact it is important to review them briefly as the basis for the newer health benefit products being offered through the internet. Like MSAs, HCRAs are personal accounts funded with tax-free contributions that an individual uses to pay health care bills. Unlike MSAs however, HCRAs have traditionally been used in a secondary role to pay for co-pays, deductibles and services not covered by primary, low-deductible insurance. Also, with HCRAs the individual loses any money left in the account at the end of the year. The use it or lose it incentive of HCRAs differs from the "save it for later' incentive of MSAs Currently, a key advantage associated with an HCRAs is its flexibility relative to an MSA. This is one reason some E-benefits companies are using HCRAs as the foundation of their online health benefit products.

COMPRHENSIVE INDIVIDUAL MEDICAL ACCOUNT

A Comprehensive Individual Medical account (CIMA) is an individual health benefits account that a person uses to buy health insurance as well as to pay bills for Individual health services. This approach differs from MSAs and traditional HCRAs which are only used to pay bills for individual health care services—not the insurance policy which is provided separately. CIMAs are flexible. An individual can use a CIMA to purchase full health insurance from a health plan that has an established network of providers by combining multiple subcapitation payments and multiple contracts. With subcapitation contracts, each provider is paid a monthly fixed amount to provide only the care that the employee needs from the provider. Finally an individual can use a CIMA to simply pay all their health bills on a fee for service basis with no insurance function.

Many employers are investigating individual health benefit accounts with defined contributions, including Medical Savings Accounts, Health Care Reimbursement Accounts, and Comprehensive Individual Medical accounts. Advocates see them representing the dawn of a new era in health benefits that will empower patients and physicians while containing costs. Opponents revile them as a misguided attack on the sick and the poor. While these accounts were possible under existing law before the new health care law (PPACA) They have not found a significant place in US health care policy or health care thinking. Employers do not have confidence in their ability to control costs now or in the near future. Large employers have more weapons at their disposal than small ones who are more likely to offer only one type of health plan. About six in ten firms shop for a new plan or new insurer each year. Simply switching plans is often the cost control strategy of last resort for many firms. The Kaiser Report shows the percentage of our national health care bill paid for by government growing from 45% in 2010 to a projected 49% in2020. Even more interesting the share of health spending financed by the Federal government will go from 29% in2010 to 31% in 2020, which means that there will not be a federal take-over of the health care system.

The Single Payer Approach for Universal Health Care Coverage

The question is often asked "What if everyone had Medicare? The Census Bureau released its annual report(2011) on income, poverty, and health insurance coverage in the United States and its no surprise to learn that we are in bad shape. The number of people living in poverty was 43.6 million (14.3 percent).up sharply from 2008 and real per capita income declined 1%. There was a dramatic spike in the uninsured to a record 50.7 million in spite of the expansion of government health insurance rolls by nearly 6 million. Private health insurance coverage dropped to the lowest level since comparable data were first collected in 1987. Those who look to new health reform law, the "Patient Protection and Affordable Care Act" for a solution will be disturbed. 'PPACA' was not designed to provide universal coverage. In fact, if the new law works as planned there will still be 23 million uninsured. The consequence of being uninsured can be lethal. Research published in2010 shows about 45,000 deaths annually can be linked to a lack of coverage. That number is probably higher now. As Don McCanne, senior health policy fellow at Physicians for a National Health Program, has observed PPACA is an under-insurance program. Employers, seeing seeing little relief will expand the present trend of shifting more insurance and health care costs onto employees.

Individuals buying plans in the new insurance exchanges (which won't start till 2014) will discover that subsidies are inadequate to avoid financial hardship. Inevitably they will end up with underinsurance, spotty coverage and high deductibles. Workers who are unemployed or without employment-based insurance will move into Medicaid. (Medi-Cal in California), where providers(doctors) are reimbursed at such low rates that many will not accept patients. When congress passed the new law, it based its decision on a faulty assumption that the rest of the population will have sustainable private health insurance. But between 2008 and 2009 the number of people covered by private insurance decreased from 201 million to 194 million and the number covered by employment-based insurance declined from 176.3 million to 169.7 million. If this trend continues, as it is bound to do under present conditions the ranks of the uninsured will expand, and the new law will fall far short of the mark—cost will exceed projections or coverage will need to be reduced. Improved Medicare for all, by replacing a dysfunctional patchwork of private insurance with a single, streamlined system of financing would save about $400 billion annually in unnecessary paper work and bureaucracy. That's enough to cover all of those now uninsured and to provide every person in the United States with quality, comprehensive coverage. A single-payer plan would also furnish us with effective cost controls like the ability to negotiate fees and medications in bulk. It would permit patients to go to the doctor and hospital of their choice.

Short of a national single-payer plan, some states are eyeing a state-based single payer plan. The new law allows states to experiment with different models of reform, but not until 2017.

The Deficit Commission has marked Medicare and Medicaid as potential targets for lowering the federal deficit. They are reportedly considering at least three possibilities

- Shifting more seniors into Medicare Advantage
- Shifting more of the cost onto the individual through higher co-pays and deductibles
- Switching to a voucher program for the purchase of private insurance

These approaches would be misguided, ineffective and harmful. These are necessary social programs and are not the causes of our soaring healthcare costs, but are the result of the lack of a rational health care system.

- Medicare, which currently covers 43.4 million people accounts for 13% of total federal outlays (FY 2010) and Medicaid accounts for 8 percent.
- Medicare and Medicaid account for a much smaller proportion of our GDP (<5%) than do our other health care costs and they are rising at a slower rate.

The most effective way to controlling rising health care costs would be to address the underlying causes namely the corporatization of health care and the lack of health planning.

- Shifting more seniors into Medicare Advantage will increase federal spending because these are for profit organizations with higher administrative costs, currently 14% higher than traditional Medicare.
- Shifting more of the cost of health care onto individual Medicare beneficiaries through increased co-pays and deductibles or by changing to a voucher system will reduce federal spending with deleterious effects on the health of seniors.
- Increasing co-pats and deductibles will place increased financial strain on seniors already burdened with high out-of-pocket costs. Seniors earning less than 200% of the Federal Poverty Level spend 22% of their income on health care. Those with incomes between 200 and 400% of FPL spend an average of 15% of their income on health care.
- A recent article in the New England Journal of Medicine documents that raising Medicare HMO co-pays and deductibles results in fewer outpatient visits and more hospital admissions. It is reasonable to expect that any savings will be offset by hospital costs and may lead to poorer health results.
- Converting Medicare from a defined benefit program to a defined contribution program in which seniors are given vouchers to purchase insurance also seeks to shift more of federal health care spending onto the individual. This will likely increase total health spending.
- Single-payer supporters know that the best way to preserve and protect our American legacy, Medicare, is to improve it and expand it to everyone. Everyone in, nobody out.
- It is important to understand that health care costs per capita in the United States are the highest in the world and these are due in large part to the use of a fragmented multi-payer (multiple insurance plans). model with associated high administrative costs.
- One third of our health care dollars are used for administration rather than direct care.
- Administrative costs include developing and marketing plans, determining eligibility for the various plans and then processing the claims for the various plans each of which have different rules.
- Medicare by contrast spends less than 3% on administration.
- Every fulltime physician (in private practice).spends over $85,000 on billing and insurance functions.

- Simplifying administration by switching to a national single public fund to collect and pay out our health care dollars will save about15%, over $400 billion, of total health care spending.
- Growth of health care costs has occurred more slowly for Medicare than for private insurance.
- Financing the program with progressive taxation will amount to less than what people are paying now for premiums and out-of-pocket medical expenses.
- Using Medicare as the model and the instrument means that the authority and organization are already in place to provide all citizens with total medical care at a cost less than private care, saving physicians and hospitals the high costs of dealing with multiple private insurance companies. Choice of physician and hospital remain unchanged.
- Another important advantage to creating a single-payer national health system is that it will virtually eliminate bankruptcies due to medical debt. A study in 2009 found that 62% of personal bankruptcies in the US were due to medical costs. Nearly 80 % of those who became bankrupt due to medical costs had health insurance.
- In a single payer system, all medically necessary care is covered throughout the life of the patient.
- People pay into the system based on their ability to pay.
- There is an end to the loss of coverage with the loss of employment. there is an end to higher charges based on age, gender or medical condition.

A national single-payer health system will also help the economy

- For small businesses, single payer means relief from the increasing burden of providing health benefits to employees.
- Single payer ends job lock, providing greater security for those who may choose to open their own business.
- Single payer enables those who are staying in jobs until they are eligible for Medicare to retire early, which opens up jobs for the younger.
- By controlling health care costs single payer will allow businesses to be more competitive in the global market.

THE TAIWAN EXPERIENCE

The most recent nation to adopt a single payer health system is Taiwan in 1995. Their previous system was was one of multiple private payers and a high number of uninsured. Prior to having a national health health system only 59% of the population had health insurance and health care costs were rising by nearly 14% each year. With the new plan in place the remaining 41% had access to coverage overnight. Within nine years 99% of the people were enrolled. There was an expected bump in the first year of implementation. However within 10years health care costs had fallen from 14% to a more manageable 3.5% to 4.5% a year. Administrative costs for the system are a low 1.4%.

THE COMMONWEALTH FUND 13TH ANNUAL HEALTH POLICY SURVEY

They reviewed experiences in eleven countries focusing on access, cost and care experiences. Overall the survey found that US adults—even when insured—were the most likely to incur high medical expenses, spend more time on paper work, and have more claims denied. The countries surveyed were Australia, Canada, France, Germany, the Netherlands, New Zealand Norway, Sweden, Switzerland, the United Kingdom, and the United States.

- ➢ Twenty percent of US adults said they had serious problems paying medical bills. Responses from other countries were in the single digits. US respondents were also more likely than adults in other countries to have gone without care because of cost.
- ➢ Thirty-five percent of US adults had out-of-pocket medical spending of $1000 during the previous year, a far higher percentage than in any other country.

- When asked about access to prompt medical care, 57% of US adults said they had seen a doctor or nurse the same or next day the last time they were sick and needed care. Switzerland had the most rapid access(93%). Adults in three other countries (Canada, Norway, and Sweden) reported longer waits than US adults.
- Nearly one third of US adults (31%) reported either denial of payments by insurer or time-consuming interactions with insurers, a higher ratio than all other countries. Seventeen percent said they spent a lot of time on paperwork or disputes over medical bills, the highest rates in the survey.

SGR—The Sustainable Growth Rate

The most current threat to the Medicare system is the SGR or the Sustainable Growth Rate which refers to Medicare's physician payment system. It is a formula for total payments to physicians. In1997 congress refined the formula by which the annual change in Medicare physician fees was determined and decided that total physician payments per beneficiary should grow no faster than the economy as a whole as measured by the gross domestic product (GDP). Policy makers were concerned about increases in the volume of services that beneficiaries need since total spending equals price times volume of services. In the congressional budget process if volume grew more quickly, fees would grow more slowly or be reduced. Volume of services as well as volume of patients did grow and reimbursements to physicians have been under pressure ever since. Each year congress has had to address an automatic reduction in fees to physicians. This year the imminent reduction was 21%. Medicare's physician payments already trail those from private insurers. There is already a widespread consensus that the relative fees in the current system are a significant cause of the growing imbalance in supply of primary care and specialty services in the US health care system. That imbalance is widely perceived as a major cause of both excessive costs and inadequate quality of care. The Medicare Resource Based Relative Value Scale is used by most private insurers to determine relative prices for physicians. The expectation that total physician spending could be kept to such a low level is undoubtedly unrealistic since few countries have ever attained that target. The SGR framers were pursuing a broader agenda of trying to drive the entire Medicare system away from fee for service toward private capitated plans. If actual spending in a given year exceeds that year's target the following year's spending is supposed to be reduced proportionately, but if that reduction is insufficient then additional reductions must come in the future. Every time Congress postpones a formula-determined fee reduction, it compounds the difference between actual and expected fees, making the eventual adjustment that much more severe. The country's long term budgetary status is a serious problem, but everyone agrees that reducing Medicare's physician fees by 21% in perpetuity might create access problems for some beneficiaries and probably will hurt providers if they are especially dependent on Medicare revenues. The act of reducing physician reimbursement for services delivered seems to occur annually. As Medicare recipients increase in number and Medicare reimbursement fees are normally lower than private insurance fees, SGR becomes a threat to physicians income unless congress intervenes. Congress has intervened a number of times to preserve access to medical care for Medicare especially for office visits without procedures. This is one of the glaring problems in the Medicare payment system that needs correction. Let us not be victims of excessive number of procedures and tests if payments to physicians are not appropriate or force the physician to terminate private practice for the world of salaried positions.

The Single Payer Plan— A Possible Solution

A perusal of the health care plans of advanced industrialized countries such a we have done at the first part of this discourse reveals that most have instituted some form of government sponsored single payer plan. By this we mean the government is the responsible provider of and payer for health care. Medicare in this country is an example of single payer system. It provides a reimbursement method for all services by eligible providers such as doctors, hospitals, clinics, emergency services, nurse practitioners and physician assistants. This requires a complex managerial staff at the central level that can reimburse for services and also control quality as well as reasonable availability of quality care on the local level. It will be most popular if there is free choice of doctor and hospital though managed care programs have been instituted with success in recent years. Of special importance to many people will be the prompt availability of services without the delays or waiting times for surgery or diagnostic services. The so-called single-payer plan must also deal with congress for appropriations so cost control and budget limitations would be part of the reality of single payer health care. We have seen the development of single payer systems of health care systems in a number of European countries, as well as in Canada, Australia, Japan, Sweden, Norway and several others. Canada and Great Britain are often held up as very successful and popular programs that the US might emulate. They are both countries with very high standards in medical care, and the institutions that support it and have contributed mightily to the history of achievement in the growth of medical sciences. A look at the Canadian system as an example of a single payer system that has been operating long enough to have reliable statistics and gauge its popularity as well as faults.

Canada is more similar to the United States than any other country They are both Anglo-Saxon countries with a similar history and the same language. Although smaller in population (33 million versus 300 million) Their populations are heterogeneous including a minor percentage that are foreign borne. Since passage of the Canada Health Act in the 1970s, that nations health statistics have become increasingly superior.

Taxes and Finances: From a financial and economic standpoint there are also a number of similarities. The two countries' tax structures are similar: 36% of revenues raised come from personal income taxes in both countries and the and the highest tax rate for personal income is 46% in Canada and 44% in the United States. The percentage from social security taxes is similar as well—17% in Canada and 21% in the United States. Approximately 10-11% is raised from corporate taxes in both countries and maximum corporate tax rates are also similar 36% in Canada and 39% in the US. The percentage of gross pay going to disposable income after taxes and social transfers is somewhat higher in the United States (89%) than in Canada (76%).

Health Systems: When it comes to health systems there are both similarities and differences. In the United States in 2007 there were 2.4 physicians per 1000 population compared with Canada's ratio of 2.2 per 1000 population. In the United States there are 50% more specialists than primary care physicians, compared with 10% more specialists in Canada. In 2007 Canada had 99 general physicians and 94 specialists per 100,000 population. Comparable figures for the United States are 100 general physicians (including family physicians, general pediatricians, general internists and obstetrician/ gynecologists) and 207 specialists per 100,000 population. Medical Education systems are similar though some Canadian medical schools require only two years of university education. All are accredited by the Joint Liaison Committee on Medical Education which also accredits US medical schools. Canadian and US medical school curricula are virtually identical as are the characteristics of residency programs. In the early 1990s half of Canadian graduates went into family medicine, but this percentage declined to 32% by 2004. Canada's health care system has a strong federal structure but also allows considerable flexibility in health policy at the provincial and territorial levels. Before the 1950s Canada's health care system resembled that of the United States today. Canada's health current system can be traced to reforms enacted in Saskatchewan in 1947 when publicly administered hospital insurance was introduced. One by one the other provinces followed. By 1972 the advantages of such coverage were sufficiently well accepted that it led to the passage of the Canada Health Act. Which made universal coverage available to all citizens. Canada's national health care system included features that offered strong support for primary care—for example, no copayments for primary care visits, coupled with incentives to seek comprehensive care from generalists. In Canada private health insurance for medical care services is not permitted for services covered by the governmental health insurance which covers hospital, ambulatory, and nursing home care. The Canada Health Act mandates that all necessary care be provided without charge to patients. Pharmaceuticals, private rooms in hospitals, dental care, home care, physiotherapy and chiropractic care are not covered by the act.

Public Insurance Plans: These are administered by ten provincial and three territorial governments which may add services to those covered by the national government. Consolidated government financing of health comes partly from the federal government which has decreased its share of the funding from 25.2% in 2005 to 21.4% in2009. The remainder is generated by provincial and local governments though a variety of taxes. Details of administering public health plans are set by the provincial governments and vary across provinces. There are major differences from one province to another in who qualifies for admission to a nursing home. Prescription drug benefits also vary, as provinces can set their own payment rates and policies regarding such issues as generic drugs and deductibles or copays.

Practices and Health Centers in Canada: As in most countries, private practitioners and specialized health centers continue to exist. The Canada Health Act prohibits these doctors and clinics from participating in the governmental insurance plan if they accept private insurance for covered services. Most hospitals and nursing homes are government financed but operated by community and regional boards. Ambulatory services are provided by physicians who bill primarily by fee-for-service with rates set by negotiation with provincial medical associations. In Canada this is called the assessment fee system. Specialists are paid more for a visit made on referral—paid through consultation fees—than for a non-referral visit. This is used as a deterrent to direct access to specialists for services that should be provided in primary care. In 2005 the Supreme Court in Quebec ruled for a physician who argued that prohibiting private insurance jeopardizes the wellbeing of people urgently needing treatment. Since then the provincial government of Quebec decided to pay for key procedures, operations, and certain tests such as mammography in private centers. This situation is in flux as other provinces contemplate similar action.

Costs: The administrative simplicity of the Canadian national health insurance has been partly responsible fo much lower costs for health care in Canada. These costs have been approximately $2500 less per person per year than in the United States. Growth rate in Canada for health care is about 3.5% per year whereas in the US it is about 5%. The system enjoys the support of the vast majority of Canadian citizens.

Availability of Services: Canadians have more choice in access to providers and services. There are no restrictions on Canadians' choice of physicians or hospitals whereas Americans are often restricted in such choices by the terms of their insurance plans. Although the system provides incentives to use primary care physicians, patients can see any physician on referral as well as directly. In contrast, 40% of Americans report difficulties in seeing a specialist or long waiting times to see one. Although there is a much greater supply of the most sophisticated technology, such as magnetic resonance imaging (MRI) in the United States than in Canada, waiting times for such diagnostic services are relatively short. For any technical service needed but not available, the patients are referred to the United States with reimbursement by Canadian health insurance. There is little elective use of US services by Canadians and no co-payments to deter use. In the United States low-income people have many fewer visits to a physician than wealthier people. However in Canada, the differences between income groups are smaller. Part of this is the result of the absence of co-pays and a better distribution of primary care physicians. There are differences by education level in the use of specialist visits. Canada has better rankings than the United States for major indicators in ten of the 12 indicators used to compare industrialized countries. Canada ranked 3rd behind the United States and Germany in cost of care. OECD(Organization for Economic Cooperation and Development) data shows that Canadians are on average healthier than Americans with lower mortality, mobility limitations, obesity, hypertension, diabetes, and respiratory disorders. The United States does marginally better on 5 year survival from cancer. Survival of poor people in Canada is better than in the United States for both African Americans and white populations and better survival among lower income Canadians than among lower-income Americans. Canada achieves the three structural characteristics of good health systems,—such as the extent of population coverage, the cost of premiums, and the supply of primary care physicians at the state level. The US does not. Canada's efforts to distribute resources equitably have been more successful than in the United States but are less adequate than than other countries such as Sweden, Finland, Denmark, The Netherlands, Spain, and the United Kingdom. In 2007 fewer than one in eight Canadians believed that their health system needed rebuilding compared with more than one in three in the United States. There are few differences in accessibility to primary care among those with insurance in the United States and Canada whereas there is greater accessibility to specialist care in the United States.

Declines in the primary care workforce in Canada are being addressed. The effort includes reallocation of funds to increase the number of instructional hours for family physicians in the first two years of postgraduate training and to provide for family medicine support groups. In contrast the United States continues to follow a long pattern of rising production of specialists with falling supplies of primary care physicians. The United States is the only OECD country to lack a universal publicly accountable health insurance system and the only one to rely on employer-based health insurance for the non-elderly population. France protects patients with chronic illnesses from co-insurance fees. Germany does not impose cost sharing for preventive services for children. Germany also limits co-pays to 1-2 % of annual income for people with chronic illnesses and low income. Both Australia and New Zealand require copayments with exceptions for some low income patients The Netherlands, New Zealand and the United Kingdom require patients to register with a general practitioner who acts as a gatekeeper to specialists. The pharmaceutical process is stronger in Canada than in the United States by virtue of reviewing both the clinical and cost-effectiveness of drugs compared with alternative therapy. Canada's experiences show these critical features of health systems can be achieved in the context of a federal structure with decentralized administrative control. Canada has achieved better health levels than the United States and the gap has widened over time.

We should take note of a move by the Ontario government to reduce the excessive retail prices of generic drugs in Canada. The Ontario government effectively halved the rate of reimbursement of ingredient costs and banned the professional allowances or kick-backs paid to pharmacies by generic manufacturers. Tax payers and private payers will save hundreds of millions of dollars. Pharmacies had previously been receiving 50% of the price of the corresponding branded and originally patented drug and henceforth they would receive only 25%. The gainers of this policy change are Ontario taxpayers, patients and (eventually).privately insured workers and their employers. Patients benefit immediately, taxpayers gain as the debt burden is reduced and workers/employers will gain if and when private insurance premiums fall. Investors in Pharmaceutical companies and pharmacies will lose. Other provinces are following Ontario's lead.

The Canadian system while popular with the people was not always popular with the doctors who feared for their income. As a matter of fact the doctors went on strike twice in the history of development of the present provincial system and lost both times. Canadian doctors were always well paid. Over 60 years, into the 21st century physician income grew at a rate of increase that outpaced that of other Canadians. Since 1958 through the advent of Medicare until at least 1992 and probably into the present, physicians as a professional category, were the top earners in the country. Compared with US doctors Canadian physicians have almost always earned less. Canadian physicians earned proportionately most in the early years of Medicare peaking around 1972 when amounts equaled and briefly exceeded US medical income.

An analogy can be found here with the apparent boom in US medical income associated with the advent of US Medicare in 1965. A 1990 study showed that although per capita expenditures on health in the United States were higher than those in Canada the actual number of services were lower. Canadian citizens were getting more and spending less. Real data on the income of physicians is hard to come by. More importantly, real data on 'take home' pay after all expenses are paid is very difficult to obtain. Still physician income is an important attraction for undertaking the long and difficult training that is required and could influence the supply dynamics.

Alternative Plans— State-Based Single Payer Health Care in Vermont

It is well known that administrative costs in the fragmented medical insurance system in the US are responsible for upwards of 30% of US medical care expenses under the present system. In addition to this the paper work required of physician offices dealing with 200 insurance plans requires a large expensive staff of billing clerks to process claims. Every insurance company has its own paperwork, payment schedules, and policies about what it will cover. Money spent on such overhead does not go towards improving patient care. Sometimes the amount of time a doctor spends on paperwork equals the amount of time spent on patient care. The state of Vermont has been active in designing and developing a publicly financed medical system that would deliver medical benefits to every resident of the state. A large part of the paper work is not in reference to patient care but to what insurance plans allow or don't allow. Psychiatric patients may not get to see a doctor if there is not a provider in network. Diagnostic tests to follow up treatments may be denied. Some just give up practicing medicine because of the hassle.

William C. Hsiao, PH.D. was asked by the state of Vermont to design a single payer system of healthcare because the status quo in health care has become untenable. Despite numerous reforms over the past 15 years, Vermont's health care costs are escalating rapidly, straining the budget, household incomes and employers bottom line. More than 7% of citizens are uninsured and another 15% have inadequate insurance. Vermont faced a $150 million budget shortfall. Employers felt that health care costs were jeopardizing their businesses and financial viability, while families struggle to pay out of pocket health care costs. Vermonters have rich insurance benefits approaching ACA's "platinum" standards. Similarly doctors and hospitals were unwilling to accept reductions in their net incomes. He found that the system capable of producing the greatest potential savings and achieving universal coverage was a single-payer system—one insurance fund that covers everyone with a standard benefit package paying uniform rates to all providers through a single payment mechanism and claims processing system. Analysis showed that Vermont could quickly save almost 8% in health care expenditures through administrative simplification and consolidation plus another 5% by reducing fraud and abuse. He recommended that the single payer be a public-private partnership. An independent board with representation from both the major health care payers (employers, the state, and workers) and the major beneficiaries and recipient of payment (providers and consumers).would negotiate updates to the benefit package and payment rates. The system reduces the rate of cost increases over time by insulating health care spending from politics and paying providers through capitation rather than fee for service, reducing the practice of defensive medicine by implementing a no-fault medical malpractice system. He estimated that Vermont could save 25% in health care expenditures over 10 years. Eligibility for coverage in the system would be based solely on proof of Vermont residency. This approach effectively divorces health benefits from employment, however the system would be supported through a payroll contribution on all Vermont wages split between employer and employee to preserve the federal tax treatment of health benefits—a tax expenditure worth $400million to $500 million in Vermont. It was recommended to delay implementation of the single-payer system until after Vermont's insurance exchange has been operating for a year, at which point Vermont will have a basis for arguing for a waiver from ACA requirements and estimating the amount of a federal block grant it would receive before 2017, when current ACA law allows for waivers. The Governor signed Vermont's health reform bill in May, 2011.

The Netherlands Experience with Managed Competition for Medicare

The Netherlands represents an experience with regulated competition among private health insurance companies. US ideas about managed competition helped to shape health care reform in the Netherlands. In 2006, the Netherlands instituted a mandated private insurance system similar to Switzerland's. Under this reform all legal residents of the Netherlands are required to purchase basic insurance from private insurers. Private plans are heavily regulated. They cannot turn down applicants, regardless of health status, and must charge community-rated premiums. A risk equalization scheme varies payment to health plans according to their enrolled populations risk profile. This requirement was put in place to reduce plans' incentives to select profitable patients and ensure that plans with sicker, higher-cost populations are not financially penalized. Insurance plans were expected to compete on the basis of price and quality by selectively contracting with networks of hospitals, physicians and other medical care providers. In 2011, insurance premiums averaged about $1749 per person with a mandatory deductible of $248. Workers must additionally contribute earmarked payroll taxes for health insurance—7.75% of their wages up to a maximum of $3,774. General taxes also help to fund government health care expenditures, including paying all premium costs for children under the age of 18 years. A separate insurance program requiring another 12% payroll tax finances long-term care. Supplemental coverage for services such as dental care and physical therapy is purchased by about 90% of persons with basic insurance The reality of managed competition in the Netherlands has not matched the rhetoric. Four key points emerge from the Dutch experience. First Competition has not sharply slowed the rate of growth in health care spending. Health care spending continues to outpace general inflation having increased at an average annual rate of 5% since 2006. At the same time, the total costs of health insurance for Dutch families including premiums and deductibles, increased by 41%. According to Statistics Netherlands, in 2010 the country spent 14.8% of its gross domestic product on health care and welfare (including long-term care and other social services) Reforms aimed at increasing and managing competition produced high administrative costs and complexity. Administering premium subsidies for low income people has been expensive. More than 40% of Dutch families now receive such subsidies—And the national tax department hired more than 600 extra staff to check incomes each month and calculate the value of the vouchers. Secondly some Dutch people remain uninsured, and there has been a substantial increase in the number of insured persons failing to pay their insurance premiums. The number of uninsured people has decreased since 2006 from about 240,000 to 150,000 but a growing number of defaulters—319,000 in 2010—haven't paid their insurance premiums for more than 6 months. Third the expansion of consumer choice has not worked. Since 2007 only 4% of the Dutch population has changed plans each year. Currently four insurance conglomerates control 90% of the Dutch health insurance market. Fourth the Netherlands still relies heavily on and needs regulation to control and supervise insurance companies that seek to escape centralized, bureaucratic control of medical care. Insurers must offer comprehensive coverage and direct payments by patients amount to less than 10% of total medical care costs.

The myth that competition has been key to cost containment in the Netherlands has obscured a crucial reality. System wide regulation of spending rather than competition among insurers is the key to controlling health care costs. The Dutch reforms have fallen far short of expectations.

Trends and Reforms in Managed Care and Insurance Companies

Insurance companies are beginning to manage doctors and thereby health care in a more active way. The barrier between companies that provide health coverage and those that actually provide health care to patients is crumbling. United health group sells technology to hospitals and other insurers, distributes drugs, manages clinical trials and offers continuing education. United's health services is quietly taking control of doctors who treat patients covered by United's plans in several areas of the country—buying medical groups and launching physician management companies. Other large insurers including Humana and Wellpoint have announced deals involving doctors in recent months, part of a strategy to curb rising health costs that could cut into profits and to weather new challenges arising from the new federal health law. Many patients insured by these companies are going to see much tighter management of their care. Wellpoint entered the business of running clinics when it announced that it would acquire CareMore a health plan operator based near Los Angeles that owns 26 clinics. Their reasoning is "the only way to stem those rising costs in the long term is to manage care on the front end. This means enlisting doctors. Their orders drive most health care spending including such items as: treating heart patients with expensive stents when cheaper drugs might work, or overusing high-tech imaging devices. By managing doctors directly insurers believe they can reshape the practice of medicine and protect their profits. Another large insurer, Cigna, saves 9% on patients treated by doctors in a Phoenix medical group it controls. Cigna has expanded over the last months in response to the new health law and it now serves patients in 32 locations.

The insurance companies feel that the doctors are incentivized to do more tests and procedures. If the doctors are employed by a managed care company their reasoning is that they will be incentivized to do less. Profit pressure can affect care decisions but is this bad? While hospitals are widely seen as the natural leaders of ACO's (Accountable Care Organizations) United's strategy positions is to lead the new systems too.

Major U.S. health insurers, including Aetna Inc, Humana Inc, and Wellpoint Inc, are retooling to become more than just health plans, in the wake of the federal health-care overhaul that is changing the rules for the industry's core business. Diversification plans include stepped up acquisitions and partnerships that will allow the companies to employ doctors directly, deliver health information technologies and participate in new hospital-doctor groups known as accountable-care-organizations. Insurance profit margins have historically averaged 7% to 8% but the health overhaul—which requires insurers to spend more on medical care instead of profits is expected to reduce that to between 3% to 5%. Meanwhile, health IT (information technology) is growing briskly and can command fat margins because of low overhead. UnitedHealth Group is expected to earn margins of about 14% this year on its health IT business and has earned margins higher than 20% in years past according to Goldman Sachs. Managed care companies have been on buying sprees before, mostly to gobble up competing insurers, and expand their networks and membership. But with the health law stripping thick profit margins from the business of providing health care benefits, that isn't a very popular move anymore. Since 2010, about 20% of the deals by managed-care companies involved health IT firms, up from 7% in 2007, while insurers buying other insurers dropped to 27% of the deals from 39% over the same period according to FactSet Research Systems, a company that ran an analysis on the market. At Aetna the new Chief Executive is implementing a strategy that will see the Hartford, Conn company get more deeply into health-information technology and run the back-end operations of the new Accountable-Care organizations, or ACO's. In 2011 Aetna spent $500 million on a technology company, Medcity, which sells software to securely transmit health data so health-care providers with many different systems can share patient information. Health IT business is expanding due to some $27 billion in federal funding available for hospitals and doctors to computerize their records. That same year Aetna announced plans to partner with Carilion Clinic in Virginia to build an ACO—a concept outlined in the health law to make the health-care system interconnected and hold down costs. In late April the same year Aetna was buying Prodigy Health holdings for $600 million to get more deeply into the business of providing mid-sized companies with a self-funded insurance option. In the accountable-care organizations, the hospitals or doctor groups would take on some of the financial risk of caring for patients—the role traditionally played by insurance companies. Aetna hopes to provide the know-how. Even if the law is ultimately repealed, health insurers see opportunities to sell services to help improve how the health system works. Health-care reform was an action—forcing event promoting the necessity for change in the insurance business. Further in the future are plans for a health-care app store. By the end of 2011, the insurer hopes consumers will be able to download mobile applications, such as a program that could help patients find doctors. Already doctors can install CareSuite, a work-flow tool for physician offices. The tools will be available regardless of whether Aetna is their insurer.

Reinventing the health-insurance business has its challenges and also new risks. Executives feel that newer areas are growing a lot faster than the traditional core business. For instance, specialty businesses, such as stand-alone dental or vision coverage may command margins over 10%. Another possibility is to export these innovations overseas for even higher margins of profit. Michael McAllister, chief executive of Humana is getting into the business of employing doctors and is eyeing home health care because these areas are growing faster than the core business. Home health care commands margins in the mid teens and also has the advantage for an insurer of keeping patients at home instead of costly nursing facilities. Humana spent nearly $800 million to buy Concentra, which runs urgent—and occupational-clinics in about 40 states. Concentra employs about 1000 primary-care doctors who are near to where three million Humana members live. Humana hopes the centers can provide an alternative to costly emergency-room care for its members. A typical visit to a Concentra urgent-care clinic costs $190 to $200, including an x-ray, according to the company, while a comparable visit to the ER would range from $350 to $650or more with additional services for x-rays. The Concentra deal is also a way to capitalize on the looming shortage of primary-care doctors when an estimated 32 million people gain coverage in2014 due to the new health law. Meanwhile Wellpoint said it is diversifying more heavily into consumer-oriented and health IT businesses. The company plans to create a portfolio of new non-core growth businesses. Wellpoint is engaged in a range of partnership discussions with leading technology and consumer companies to redefine health IT.

ACOs: Accountable Care Organizations is a concept of health care that is very similar to the Managed Care Experiments of the 1990s that failed to achieve goals of health care at reduced cost. Providers receive a set annual payment to cover the costs of all care and get to keep whatever they don't spend on patients. The obvious business strategy is to recruit relatively healthy patients and subtle queues that those with expensive illnesses would be better off elsewhere. An ACO can game risk adjustments by eliminating additional diagnoses that would up its capitation payments and make its outcomes look better. The more expensive providers label their patients with more diagnoses. Measures of quality like death rates or community wellbeing are either too rare or too subtle for reliable statistics. Evidence from the UK shows that providers will improve on the aspects of care that are measured but neglect those that are not and its not clear that monitoring quality measures has actually improved quality or prevented abuses.

What About the VA System as a Model for Delivery of Health Care

Since the Veterans Health Administration (VHA) was engineered to follow a more decentralized managed care template more than 15 years ago it has demonstrated accumulating achievements in health and health care delivery. In chronic disease management and preventive care the VHA has surpassed Medicare, commercial managed care, and various community health systems using broadly accepted process measures. Beneficiaries of the VHA seem to have health outcomes—including mortality—that are the same as or better than those of Medicare and private sector patients These findings are noteworthy considering the population served by the VHA which is recognized to be burdened by socioeconomic disadvantage, co-morbid illness, and poor self-reported health. It is remarkable that the VHA has been able to attain this superior quality care at a lower cost than that purchased through Medicare with expenditures that have increased at a much slower rate (adjusted annual per capita growth rate, 0.3% vs 4.4%). By using process measures that reflect receipt of high quality care. Keating and colleagues compared the treatment of older male veterans in the VHA system with that of fee-for-service Medicare patients with a diagnosis of colo-rectal, lung, prostate, or hematologic cancer. They found that patients treated in the VHA system had higher rates of curative resection for colon cancer, and recommended chemotherapeutic regimens for hematologic neoplasms, and biphosphonate use for multiple myeloma. The authors use state-of-the-art statistical methods to address the issue of differences in settings and patient populations. They adjusted for characteristics such as age, race, and region that could have a confounding effect. The only process measure for which the VHA patients had lower scores than Medicare patients was the use of 3-dimensional conformal radiation therapy versus intensity-modulated external-beam radiation therapy for prostate cancer. This divergence may reflect varying adoption rates of new technology by 2 distinct health care financing schemes, highlighting the difference between the market driven practices of the fee-for-service sector and the careful consideration given to large capital investments required of a system that must adhere to an annual budget. If we ever hope to control health care costs as providers and as a nation, policies to encourage high quality evidence of benefit before rapid dissemination of novel technologies, especially expensive ones, are needed both in the VHA and Medicare settings. Despite the clamor of special interest groups, corporate lobbying, and American distaste for government-run institutions, the public option may yet find its voice in the latest accomplishments demonstrated by the VHA. Considering the possible repeal of the Patient Protection and Affordable Care Act there is reason to celebrate the triumphs of the country's largest integrated and publicly funded health care network. This is an example of a single payer system in the US that works and works well. It provides good if not better health care for the veteran population and is available in all states through a system of clinics and hospitals that are made convenient to all those that are eligible. This is a tax payer financed system while not completely free is certainly affordable.

Drugs and the Drug Companies

There is more to health care than access to a doctor or a hospital. The expansion of health care givers such as nurse practitioners and physician assistants add to our access to health care and also to the cost. High tech devices in hospitals and offices also play a significant role in the cost increases we have experienced. Another less known factor is the cost and indeed the availability of drugs and medicines of all descriptions. This is important because we already pay on average about twice the cost per capita for health care than other industrialized countries. At the present time and in the recent past costs for delivery of health care have been rising 5% to 7% a year. How long this country can continue to support this kind of economic burden is a question that a bankrupt government will have to answer. Back to the question of drugs and pharmaceutical companies. Multinational big Pharma charges the American public the highest pharmaceutical prices in the world while it sells the same drugs all over the world at one-half, one-third or even one tenth of the price they charge in the United States. They do this because in the rest of the industrialized world there is legislation that limits profits for medications, while the U.S. allows these companies to charge whatever the market will bear. The Affordable Care Act does not address this issue. Himmelstein and Woolhandler have recommended amongst other things that we eliminate: Medicare Advantage Plans; Give Medicare the power to negotiate drug prices; Eliminate private Part D plans which have high overhead and replace them with a public drug benefit along traditional Medicare principles; Ban participating physicians from prescribing medications or medical devices (including orthopedic and cardiac implants).produced by device or drug makers from whom they receive payments; Reduce fees paid to the highest paid specialists, generally those who prescribe or use expensive drugs and devices.

There are other issues involving drug companies that should be mentioned since they involve cost and availability of essential drugs. William Faloon of Life Extension Magazine has pointed out that drug manufacturers have been known to inflate drug prices by frivolous lawsuits against generic drug makers in order to delay approval of a lower-cost generic and continue to earn millions by the delay. There is profit to be made for each extra day that its expired-patent drug retains market exclusivity. Apparently the filing of law suites against generic manufacturers for the purpose of delaying FDA approval has gone on for years. Once the Generic maker defeats the imaginary claims, it then has to charge more to the consumer because of the millions of dollars it was forced to squander on legal fees. This is one reason why generics cost more than they should. The FDA and Congress have not addressed this ongoing problem. As an example of what a pharmaceutical firm has done to retain and promote a lucrative product from going to the generic market is the maneuvering by Sanofi to keep its brand name product Lovenox, a low-molecular weight heparin drug, with sales over $4billion in 2009, that was about to lose its patent protection. Sanofi first tried to hold off generic competition by filing a suit in federal court to block FDA approval of generic versions made by other companies but failed in two court cases. Sanofi then filed a safety petition alleging that it was against the public interest to allow a low-cost generic to be sold. Sanofi urged doctors and medical associations to contact the FDA and express concern about the safety of generic versions of the drug when this was not successful it used payments of almost $5million dollars to influence groups to contact the FDA and support its petition, all of this to argue and express concern about the safety of generic Lovenox. None of the organizations or person that received the large donations disclosed to the FDA that they had been paid by Sanofi to support the lucrative Lovenox monopoly and mislead the FDA at the expense of Medicare, Medicaid, and health insurance premium payers. There are other examples of cover-ups such as the suicide rate associated with Chantix a brand name drug made by Pfizer and the current shortage of many life saving drugs. A shortage means higher prices. By midyear 2011 a record-breaking 180 different drugs needed to treat leukemia, solid tumors, infections and other diseases were declared in short supply. In2010 two patients died because the hospital could not get morphine and substituted a more powerful drug. Another instance a patient died when a drug in short supply (epinephrine) had to be diluted so much it was ineffective. A fourth patient died because they could not get the appropriate antibiotic to treat the infection. Chemotherapy sessions were postponed because necessary drugs were not available. The underlying reasons for most of these drug shortages is pharmaceutical profits. In some cases soon after a shortage new supplies become available at prices as much as 20 times higher than before the shortage occurred.

In other cases doctors are forced to use expensive brand-name drugs because low-cost generics disappeared from the market. Sometimes pharmaceutical companies will say that the cost of older products no longer justifies making them. The FDA regulations can be serious stumbling blocks for manufacturers to start producing drugs that are needed. One solution being proposed is to create a federal government-funded stockpile of crucial cancer medicines to overcome a problem created by regulations. A group of oncologists has started a non-profit drug company to import drugs from other countries. If there were no artificial barriers (regulations) erected against imported drugs there would be no shortages, as there are ample supplies of these medications in other countries. As of last summer, of 34 generic cancer drugs on the market, 14 were in short supply. These include mainstay treatments for leukemia, lymphoma, and testicular cancer. Oncologists are being forced to use newer brand-name drugs that don't have a proven cure rate but can cost 100 times more than the effective generics that are in short supply. Unscrupulous wholesalers may offer drugs in short supply at prices that are 10 to 20 times the normal rate. Such sales may be legal but now we have problems that overbearing regulations were enacted to prevent. Clinical trials of new drugs are postponed because studies must also offer older medicines that cannot be reliably provided. In spite of overpricing the United States faces an unprecedented shortage of prescription medications. These are probably the results of over regulation of medicine by our political leaders.

Research by Physicians for a National Health Program

Over the past two decades, PNHP has 'framed' the debate and focused it on the need for fundamental health care reform. Some of these findings have become well known and are summarized thusly.

- Administrative costs consume 31 percent of US health spending, most of it unnecessary. The US could save enough on administrative expenses (nearly $400 billion).annually with a single payer to cover all the uninsured.
- Nearly 45,000 Americans die each year for lack of health insurance. The uninsured do not receive all the medical care they need—they live sicker and die younger. Those most in need of preventive services are least likely to receive them.
- Medical bills contribute to more than 60% of all bankruptcies. Three-fourths of those bankrupted had health insurance at the time they got sick.
- Taxes already pay for over 60 percent of US health spending. Americans pay the highest health care taxes in the world. We pay for national health insurance but don't get it.
- Despite spending far less per capita for health care, Canadians are healthier and have better measures of access to health care than Americans.
- Business pays less than 20 percent of our nations health bill. It is a misnomer that our health system is 'privately financed' (60percent is paid by taxes and the remaining 20 percent is out-of-pocket payments)

- For-profit, investor-owned hospitals, HMOs and nursing homes have higher costs and score lower on most measures of quality than their non-profit counterparts.
- Immigrants and emergency department visits by the uninsured are not the cause of high and rising health care costs.
- Computerized medical records and chronic disease management do not save money. The only way to slash administrative overhead and improve quality is with a single payer system.
- Alternative proposals for "universal coverage" do not work. State health reform efforts over the past two decades have failed to reduce the number of uninsured.

Uninsured and Underinsured in the United States

The number of Americans without health insurance jumped by 2.2 million to 47 million (15.8 percent of the population) in 2006. They are estimated to number about 50 million now in 2012. The proportion of people covered by employer-sponsored private coverage fell from 69 percent in 2000 to 59 percent in 2006. Government employees account for about one-fourth of all people with employer sponsored coverage. The number of uninsured children rose by 611,000 to 8.7 million in 2006, 11.7 percent of all children. With private employer-sponsored coverage deteriorating rapidly the number of uninsured children has fallen only 17 percent since SCHIP was enacted in 1997, from 10.7 million to 8.66 million. Over 6.6 million were covered by SCHIP in 2006.

15.3 million Hispanics (34.1 percent) were uninsured in 2006 up 1.3 million from 2005. 7.6 million Blacks (20.5 percent) were uninsured in 2006, up 600,000 from2005. In Massachusetts, often cited as a model for health reform, the number of uninsured increased from 583,000 in2005 (9.2 percent). to 657,000 in 2006(10.4 percent)

90.9 million Americans (30.6 percent) were covered by government programs or the VA in 2006. This included 40.3 million people with Medicare (13.6 percent), 38.3 million with Medicaid (12.9 percent) 10.6 million 3.6 percent) with VA/military and 1.7 million in other programs (under 1 percent) (United States Census Bureau)

Almost 40 million (20 percent) Americans can't afford or access needed health care according to a report from Centers for Disease Control and Prevention (CDC). One fifth of Americans can't afford one or more of the following services: medical care, prescription medicines, mental health care, dental care, or eye glasses. (Centers for Disease Control and the National Center for Health Statistics).

In 2009 a record 50.7 million Americans (16.7 percent).including 7.5 million children, were uninsured up from 46.3 million (15.4 percent).in2008. The huge increase in Americans lacking health coverage was almost entirely due to a sharp decline in the number of people with employer-based coverage, down 6.6 million since 2008. Since 2000, employer-based coverage has plummeted from 64.2 percent of the population to 55.8 percent. The increase in uninsured would have been much higher had there not been a huge expansion of public coverage, primarily Medicaid to an additional 5.8 million people last year (2010). Medicaid now covers more than 48 million people, a record 15.7 percent of the population.(US census Bureau 2010)

63 million Americans (19.8 percent) were uninsured for at least part of 2010, up from 58.5 million people in2009(National Center for Health Statistics). There was a slight drop in the number of uninsured children as public programs for children, primarily Medicaid and CHIP continued to expand. Still 8.7 million children were uninsured for at least part of 2010. (National Health Interview Survey, 2010, June 2011). Nine million working-age Americans who had health insurance through a job that was lost—became uninsured between 2008 and 2010, according to a survey by the Commonwealth Fund. Among those who lost employer-sponsored coverage only 25% were able to find another source of coverage and only 1 in7 were able to retain their job-based coverage through COBRA. In 2010 75 million adults went without necessary health care due to cost, 73 million reported having trouble paying bills, or were in medical debt, and 29 million used up all their savings to pay medical debt. A quarter of adults with chronic conditions skipped prescriptions due to cost. One third of people under 65 who are diagnosed with cancer are uninsured during or after diagnosis, with 75% reporting that their lack of coverage is due to high premiums costs or a pre-existing condition exclusion (American Cancer Society, "A National Poll: Facing Cancer in the Health Care System, 2010). A cancer diagnosis is also a risk factor for personal bankruptcy. In Washington State they found that in a registry of 231,799 cancer cases, 2.1 % sought personal bankruptcy protection in the years following the diagnosis. For example, five years after receiving a diagnosis of lung cancer, 7.7 % of victims sought bankruptcy (Rachel Feinzeig, "Study Illuminates Link between Cancer, Bankruptcy," Wall Street Journal Blog Bankruptcy Beat, 6/7/11)

The number of hospital emergency departments (EDs) in non-rural areas declined 27% between 1990 and 2007. Safety-net hospitals, hospitals in counties with a high poverty rate and for-profit hospitals with low profitability or located in highly competitive markets were more likely to close their EDs.

The economic crisis has hit Hispanic and black households the hardest. Between 2005 and 2009 the median wealth of Hispanic households dropped by 66%, compared to a 53% drop in median wealth of black households and a 16% drop among non-hispanic white households. The decline has led to the largest wealth disparities in the 25 years that the Census Bureau has been collecting data. Health-care premiums will rise 8.5% in 2012 according to a Price-Waterhouse suvey of 1700 firms. Employers are offering workers more meager plans in response to higher costs: 17% of employers surveyed most commonly offered high-deductible health plans to their workers this year, up from 13% in 2010(Merrill Goozner, The Fiscal Times, 5/18/11)

US health expenditures in 2011are projected to be $2.7 trillion, $8,649 per capita, 17.7per cent of GDP. Over the next decade, health spending is predicted to grow 5.8% annually. In 2020, after the Patient Protection and Affordable Care Act is fully implemented health spending is projected to be $4.6 trillion, $13, 709 per capita, 19.8 per cent of GPD (Office of the Actuary, National Health Spending Projections through 2020, Health Affairs, July 28, 2011.)

Starbucks spent over $250 million on health insurance for its US employees in 2010 more than it spent on coffee(Jennifer Haberkorn, "Starbucks CEO rethinks health law", Politico, 03/22/11)

The total cost of health care for a family of four covered by a preferred provider plan (PPO) in 2011 is estimated to be $19,393, up 7.3 per cent from 2010 according to the Milliman Medical Index. Employer contributions account for 59%, $11,385 of the total, while employees pay 41 percent of the cost, $8,008. On average employees will contribute $4,728 to premiums and pay $3,280 in out-of-pocket costs. (DON McCanne, "The Milliman Medical Index, 5/12/11) The average cost of employer-sponsored health coverage rose 5percent to $13,770($1,147 per month) for family coverage and $5,049 ($421 per month) for individual coverage) in 2010. The cost of employer-sponsored coverage has more than doubled since 2000 (Employer Health Benefits Annual Survey, 2010, Kaiser Family Foundation)

Medicaid spending is set to decline for only the second time in the program's 46 year history as additional federal funding from the 2009 economic stimulus package dries up as of July 2011. Medicaid spending was up 8.2 per cent to $354 billion in 2010 due to a 14.2 per cent increase in federal funding. With enrollment expected to grow 6.1 percent in the coming year due to the continued economic downturn, 24 states are planning to cut payments to providers and 20 states are planning to cut benefits. Medicaid currently consumes about 22 per cent of state budgets. (Robert Pear," As Number of

Medicaid Patients Goes Up, Their Benefits Are About to Drop." The New York Times 06/15/ 11)

Florida's disastrous experience with for-profit Medicaid managed care in the 1990's (when up to 50% of funding was diverted to over head and profits by unscrupulous firms) has not deterred Florida's legislators from again pushing for privatization of the state's Medicaid program, claiming it will control costs. In fact, per capita Medicaid spending rose more slowly between 2001and 2009 than spending on private coverage by large employers (up 30 per cent vs 112per cent, respectively).(Greg Mellowe, Florida Center for fiscal and Economic Policy 4/1/11: investigative reporters Fred Schulte and Jenni Bergal published a series of articles on fraud in Florida's 1990s Medicaid managed care programs in the Florida Sun Sentinel). Children with Medicaid coverage are much more likely to be denied treatment or made to wait long periods for an appointment with medical specialists. Across eight different specialties, 66per cent of children with Medicaid were denied an appointment at a doctor's office compared to 11 per cent with private coverage. In clinics that accepted both, the average wait time for an appointment was 22 days longer for a child with Medicaid compared to one covered by private insurers. The study increased concern about the quality of care under the Affordable Care Act, which relies heavily on Medicaid expansion to increase coverage nationwide, (Bisgaier and Rhodes, "Auditing Access to Specialty Care for Children with Public Insurance", NEJM, 6/16/11.)

MEDICARE: Administrative costs for Medicare were 1.4 percent in 2008, excluding overhead in private Medicare Advantage and Part D pharmaceutical plans, according to the 2010 Medicare Trustees Report. Medicare's administrative overhead fell slightly to 1.3 per cent in 2009. Including the overhead from private plans in Medicare's overhead raises it to 5.3 percent, the figure reported in the National Health Expenditure Accounts(2008) (CMS, 2009 and 2010 Annual Reports of the Board of Trustees).Medicare benefits are inadequate. Medicare households on average spent $4,620 on health care in 2009, more than twice what non-Medicare households spent, according to the Kaiser Family Foundation. The program for 47 million seniors and the permanently disabled currently covers less than half of the health care costs of beneficiaries who on average subsist on incomes below $22,000 a year and have less than $33,000 in retirement accounts and other savings. On top of standard premiums of $115.40 a month, enrollees pay a $1,132 deductible for each hospital stay and hundreds more for long stays. Medicare beneficiaries are also responsible for 20% of the bills for most outpatient care. Medicare doesn't cover dental, vision, hearing or long-term care, and has no cap on out-of-pocket spending. (Levy, "Making Medicare

Beneficiaries pay more" Los Angeles Times, 7/15/11) Costs for Medicare patients are being better contained than those covered under commercial insurance plans according to David Blitzer, chairman of the Standard and Poor (S&P) Index Committee Medicare spending, as measured by the S&P Medicare Index, increased by 2.8% between March 2010 and March 2011 a far lower rate of inflation than seen for private medical coverage which rose 7.6 %, according to the S&P.

CORPORATE MONEY AND CARE

US physicians spend nearly four times more on billing and insurance related overhead each year than their Canadian counterparts ($82,975 vs $22,205 per physician), with US Medical practice staff spending over 20.6 hours per week on bureaucratic tasks, compared to just 2.5 hours per physician per week under Canada's single-payer program. Morra et al, "US physician practices versus Canadians.(Health Affairs, 8/11) Seven top executives at drug, insurance, and hospital trade associations received a total of $33.2 million in compensation during the height (2008-2009) of the health care reform fight. The nation's five largest health insurers netted $ 11.7 billion in profits in 2010, up 51% from 2008, because medical costs grew slower than forecast as insured patients skimped on medical care to avoid costly co-pays and deductibles during the severe recession. United Health Care was the leader in profitability taking in over $4.6 billion in profits, followed by Wellpoint ($2.9 billion) and Aetna ($1.8 billion). Profits were up 361 percent over 2008 at Cigna, to $1.3billion in2010 and up 70% at Humana, to $1.1 billion. Meanwhile health insurers are proposing double-digit premium increases claiming the demand for medical services may surge at the end of the year(Reed Abelson "Health Insurers Making Record profits as many postpone Care" The New York Times 5/13/11) (Health Insurers Pocketed Huge Profits in 2010 Despite Weak Economy", Health Care for America Now, 3/03/11).

Seven of California's largest health insurers were fined close to 5 million dollars by state regulators in 2010 for failing to pay doctors and hospitals in a fair and timely fashion. Investigators determined that insurers paid about 80% of claims correctly, well below the legal requirement of 95%. Five of the insurers were also found to have improper provider appeals processes, sometimes requiring providers to appeal to the same person who denied their claim. Insurance companies will also be required to pay tens of millions in compensation to unpaid doctors and hospitals (Victoria Colliver, "California Largest Insurers Continue To Cheat," San Francisco Chronicle, 11/30/10).

Despite publicly claiming to support health reform and making substantial contributions to democratic politicians, the insurance industry lobbying group, America's Health Insurance Plans (AHIP) also funneled $86.2 million to the US Chamber of Commerce in 2009 to oppose the federal health law. Moreover, the nation's five largest health insurance companies have started a new coalition to lobby exclusively for their own interests and profits, independent of the small and non-profit insurers that are also represented by AHIP. The "Big Five"—Wellpoint, Unitedhealthcare, Aetna, Cigna, and Humana—have also enlisted the services of corporate public relation firms APCO Worldwide and Weber Shandwick as well as law firm Allston& Bird LLP to help craft political strategy. For starters, they seek to strip the 2010 health reform bill of provisions such as minimum requirements for the proportion of insurance premiums spent on paying for health care rather than for overhead and profit. (Drew Armstrong," Insurers Gave U.S. Chamber $86 Million Used to Oppose Obama's Health Law, Bloomberg, 11/17/10, and UnitedHealth Joins Wellpoint to Hone Health-Law Lobby", Bloomberg, 1/31/11) Indianapolis-based Wellpoint gave $450,000 to the Republican state Leadership Committee and $250,000 to the Republcan Governors Association. Wellpoint also gave $840,000 to the Repiblcan State leadership Committee for the 2010 elections (Salant, Wellpoint Joins Koch Help Fight Wisconsin State Senate Recalls., Bloomberg.com, 8/4/11).

Health insurance giants are on a buying spree for firms in health IT, physician management, and other industries that are much less regulated than health insurance and will give them an advantage in controlling health care costs according to UnitdHealth's Rick Jelinek. Since June 2009, the seven largest insurance companies have made 25 major corporate acquisitions, including only six that were health plans. In December Humana purchased Concentra, a network of urgent and occupational care centers in 40 states; over 1/3 of Humana enrollees live within 10 miles of a Concerta Clinic(Christopher Weaver," Health Insurers Respond To Reform By Snapping Up less-Regulated Businesses", Kaiser Health News, 3/19 11).

Judgments and settlements under the False Claims Act for defrauding the U.S. government have resulted in over $25 billion in repayments to the federal government since 1986 with 19 of 20 of the highest payments coming from health care corporations. In 2009, pharmaceutical giant Pfizer paid a total of $2.3 billion, including $ 1 billion under the False Claims Act and $1.3 billion as a criminal fine for paying kickbacks to physicians and other criminal offenses. Hospital chain HCA has paid $1.7 billion to the federal government, including a $ 900 million settlement in 2000 for Medicare manipulation, kickbacks, bill coding frauds, and padding. Major settlements and judgments each involving hundreds of millions of dollars, have hit the nations largest health firms including Tenet Health Care, Merck, GlaxoSmithKline, Serono, Bayer and many others (Donald R. Soeken, International Whistlblower Archive, www. whistleblowing.us). Even privately-run prisons have learned to reap profits like private insurers by cherry-picking inmates and skimping on medical care. In 2009, after adjusting for medical costs medium-security state run prisons in Arizona cost $2,834 less per prisoner than privately-run prisons (Monica Ameida "Private Prisons Found to Offer Little in Savings," The New York Times, 5/18/11)

BIG PHARMA OR THE PHARMACEUTICAL INDUSTRY

The Pharmaceutical Research and Manufacturers of America (PhRMA). lobbying group spent at least $101.2 million to influence the national health reform debate in 2009 alone. Billy Tauzin, then CEO of PhRMA, reports that spending went towards advertising," grassroots "efforts, lobbying, polling and consulting." PhRMA also donated to right-wing organizations such as the Heritage Foundation, National Review, Pacific Research Institute, and the Hudson Institute. (Bara Vaida and Christopher Weaver, "Drug Lobby's Tax Filings Reveal Health Debate Role" Kaiser Health News, 12/01/10)

Drug Companies claim to spend an average of $1.3 billion on R&D to bring a single new drug to market, but the true net median cost was closer to $59.4 million in 2000, according to a new study. The $59.4 million figure excludes research (including the cost of discovery and early development) because it cannot be accurately measured and is in any event, likely to be small for large pharmaceutical firms net of taxpayer subsidies; over 84% of all funds for discovering new medicines come from public sources. Previous research has shown that, net of taxpayers contribution drug companies spend just 1.3% of revenues on basic research to discover new molecules. Pharmaceutical R&D is increasingly churning out products ("me-too drugs").that have few benefits over existing drugs; these slightly modified drugs (copies) enable companies to profit from high-cost, patented drugs without the risks of original drug development (Light and Warburton "Demythologizing the High Costs of Pharmaceutical Research", BioSocieties 2011, and Light and Lexchin, "Foreign Free Riders and the high Price of U.S. Medicines "British Medical Journal 2005" 331.)

Novo Nordisk will pay $25 million to settle claims of illegally marketing a hemophilic drug, Factor VII, to the U.S. Army as a treatment for trauma wounds and severe bleeding,. Despite only being approved by the FDA for hemophilia treatment the military began using Factor VII (sold as NovoSeven) as a treatment for combat wounds in Iraq in2003 and it was soon adopted by trauma centers worldwide. Clinical studies have since shown that Factor VII does not control severe bleeding and can cause blood clots that lead to heart attack or stroke. In 2010, Novo Nordisk reported $1.6 billion in sales of NovoSeven, including approximately $250 million for unapproved usage. (Robert Little "Drug Maker $25 million to settle military claim.", The Baltimore Sun, 6/10/11).

The pharmaceutical industry spent $6.1 billion in2010 to influence American doctors, and another $4 billion on direct to consumer advertising, according to IMS Health. (Erica Mitrano, "Just Say No to Drug Reps." SoMdNews.com, 7/15/11).

HOSPICE, INC

For-profit hospices are expanding rapidly and may be cherry-picking the most profitable patients, according to a recent study. The number of for-profit hospices increased from 725 in 2000 to 1,660 in 2007, while the number of non-profit remained stable at 1205 in2007. Overall, 52% of facilities are for-profit, 35% are non-profit and 13% are government owned. Hospice care is funded by Medicare on a per-diem basis, with a fixed rate ($143 in 2007) paid to providers for each day that a patient is in a facility. Because the first and last days of care are more expensive to provide longer length of stay generates higher profit; The study found that patients in for-profit centers averaged a 20 day stay compared to 16 days in non-profit centers. For-profit hospices also had twice as many dementia patients compared to non-profits and had fewer cancer patients; end-of-life care is much more expensive for cancer patients than for those with dementia. An earlier study (2005) found that large investor-owned hospices generate margins nine times higher than those of large non-profits due to cherry-picking and paying lower wages and benefits to less-skilled staff. (Wachterman M W et al," Association of Hospice Agency Profit Status With Patient Diagnosis, Location of Care, and length of Stay," JAMA, Feb, 2. 2011) Hospice care costs for nursing home patients jumped nearly 70% between 2005 and 2009 from $2.5 billion to $4.3 billion while the number of hospice patients increased by only 40% according to the Office of the Inspector General(OIG). The Medicare program paid for-profit hospices more for patients than it paid non-profit and government entities in 2009. For-profit hospices received about $12,600 per patient, while non-profit and government entities received between $8,200 and $9,800 per beneficiary (Charles Fiegl, Medicare Hospice Care to Face Increased Scrutiny," Amednews, 7/28/11); DHHS Office of the Inspector General, "Medicare Hospices that focus on Nursing Facility Residents," July, 2011. For-profit hospices also provide poorer care; a full range of end-of-life services is provided half as often, and family counseling services are received only 45% as often at for profit facilities compared to non-profits. For-profit hospices are also only half as likely to provide palliative radiotherapy, a symptom relieving treatment for cancer patients. Hospice facilities are usually not chosen by the family: they are recommended by the nursing home or hospital staff. For-profit hospices also recruit patients directly from nursing homes and hospitals; Miami based VITAS Hospice Services, the largest nationwide hospice chain, pays a commission to recruiters who provide incentives to hospital and nursing home staff to refer profitable hospice patients. For-profit hospices have been indicted for paying kickbacks to medical staff for certifying patients as hospice-eligible without examining them. In 2008, Medicare expenditures on hospice exceeded $11 billion, serving more than one million patients (Marlys Harris, "The big and profitable business of dying, CBS Money Watch, 5/21/11; J Perry and R. Stone," In the Business of dying: Questioning the Commercialization of Hospice", Journal of Law, Medicine and Ethics, 5/18/11)

Spending on health Care in the U.S. in 2008 far exceeded that seen in other countries according to an analysis of health data from Australia, Canada, Denmark, France, Germany, Netherlands, New Zealand, Norway Sweden, Switzerland, the United Kingdom,. No country spent more than 70% of U.S. spending ($7,538 per capita, 16% of GDP. Despite higher spending, the U.S. ranked 6tth of the seven countries in terms of quality in a 2010 cross national study by the Commonwealth Fund with only average performance on effectiveness and patient-centeredness and low performance on safety and coordination.(David Squires," The U.S. Health System in Perspective: A Comparison of Twelve Industrialized Nations", The Commonwealth Fund, July 2011).

AN OVERALL LOOK AT A VERY COMPLICATED PROBLEM THAT MUST BE SOLVED

This odyssey through the world of health care illustrates the complexity of providing an absolute necessity for the body, mind and society as well as the culture of the country. No matter what country, color, religion, philosophy, geography or ancestral beliefs you call your own you and your family and your neighbors as well as your rulers need preventive and sick and psychiatric medical care. This applies to the poorest as well as the wealthiest and strongest country on the face of the earth. As we look at the variety of solutions or lack thereof in the world countries, we must be astonished by the variety and the complexities as well as the enormous cost of all the systems that are working or have been tried by right thinking and serious governments only to find that financial disaster threatens their very existence. On the one hand we have an item namely medical care, a rather simple concept and on the other hand we have cost and complexities of application that are baffling the best legislative and administrative minds of our times. It is obvious that we need to look to the European countries and Canada for models of universal medical care since that is the goal that all people and advanced industrialized societies seek. Simplicity is a character however that eludes the best systems that have been devised because there are so many political and financial as well as public versus private competitions for the tax and premium fee dollar. The private insurance company may be a non-profit entity in one country and a for-profit company in the next country as is the case in the United States. In some countries the system maintains both public and private hospital and clinic systems to please that portion of the citizenry that wants a private accommodation or may be unwilling to be delayed by a waiting list for diagnostic or surgical procedures. In some countries patients are required to pay a portion up front which may vary according to their income in others it is all tax supported. Some systems provide complete support for such ancillary but important services such as dental, eye examination, physiotherapy, pharmaceuticals, even holistic therapy. Most will provide emergency services like hospitalization, ambulance service, home care and preventive services such as immunization for the common childhood and elderly diseases. Would that medical care could be as simple as seeing a physician, or his nurse practitioner or his physician assistant in an office or admitted to a hospital for additional workup and treatment without the burden of cost to the patient. The real world of medicine is so much more complicated than that. We have reviewed the manpower problem that will affect delivery of medical care in the future even if you have coverage and a right to be treated without undue delay, We know that some practitioners are unable to maintain a private practice because of declining reimbursements for services from all the governmental services (Medicare and Medicaid) as well as the private insurance companies, because of the administrative burden of dealing with hundreds of insurance companies all of which have different forms, requirements, and limitations on what they will allow for billing. For the patient with private insurance in the US the out of pocket costs in the form of high deductible plans can be very high. In France a significant portion of the payment out of pocket is reimbursed but with variations based on income, age, educational status etc. In Germany everyone contributes a portion of the cost with variations. Switzerland has a variation of the non-profit insurance with deductibles. In the whole of Africa medical care exists but is a victim of desperate economic conditions. South America has a variety of systems but not universal coverage though coverage improves as the economy improves. Health care is more than having a patient, a doctor and a hospital available. Medical personnel and facilities of all types must be available and supported adequately. Declining reimbursement for physicians, nurses and other providers for the sake of insurance company profits or government budgets will result in changes in how medicine and surgery and psychiatry are practiced. We see this in the closure of private practices or early retirement. Pressure from insurance companies to reduce nursing staff or increase their load of patients or pressure to do more outpatient procedures has resulted in the loss of many nurses as well as early retirement. Doctors resent the rules imposed by insurance companies that restrict admission to a hospital, admission to an emergency room, or how long a patient can remain in the hospital irrespective of the professional opinion of the doctor. Doctors resent it when they can't earn a decent fee for a service or a procedure because the insurance company or the government agency reduces their reimbursement 20 or 30 % arbitrarily or will not allow them to raise the fee for a procedure because of rules imposed by insurance companies that are making profits in the billions and whose CEOs are receiving multimillion dollar bonuses above astronomical salaries. There are obvious reasons why medical care is so expensive in the US. Administrative costs by insurance companies in the 20-25% range account for some 400 billion dollars a year, no small sum when when administrative costs in the CMS (Medicare) are 4%. We cannot afford to support the large number of for-profit medical care insurance companies at the present level of cost to the nation and the government without going broke. We cannot afford to spend twice as much as any other industrialized nation per capita and sustain annual increases of 5 to 12 % a year.

Medical care is neither simple or cheap. It can also be very disturbing when we read about the manipulations of the markets by pharmaceutical companies to preserve or increase their profits; their restrictions on the availability of some vital drugs to manipulate prices and malfeasance perpetrated by some of our US Medical insurance companies that have resulted in millions and even billions of dollar fines.

It is time for this country to consider universal tax supported health care both as a humanitarian need and because it may be the only system we can afford to sustain. Obviously we should choose successful models that have stood the test of time and experience such as the Canadian and the United Kingdom experiences. These models must support doctors and nurses and all the other support personnel at reasonable incomes if we are to avoid shortages of these critical providers as has been predicted. If Canada can provide good professional care and services at half the capita cost why can't we. We must remember that some surgical specialties require 8 to 11 years of training and hard work. There are good reasons why many give up a career in general or cardio thoracic or neurosurgery not the least of which is the devastating experience of a malpractice suite, a very demanding life style, and declining reimbursements by government and insurance companies. There is an urgent need to reform and control the malpractice problem in this country. The threat of malpractice litigation has closed trauma centers, has denied some states OBGYN services, forced some doctors to retire early or move to a state that has instituted caps and restrictions on awards and reduced the risk and incidence of malpractice suites. It has long been said that the congress with its large number of lawyers has been reluctant to reform the litigation problem. President George Bush tried but failed. The failure to act on these problems or to take good care of our 24/7 providers may result in fewer family practitioners and surgeons and more plastic surgeons.

Peripheral Items that Need to be Considered as Part of Medical Care

There are a number of specialties and necessary services that need to be considered to some extent because they are not usually thought of in the context of doctor-patient or disease-prescription or hospitalization-surgery scenarios. But they all cost money, they are all necessary for many people at some time in their lives and would necessarily be included in any form of universal health care plan though they are not always covered even in some of our gold-plated insurance plans.

MENTAL DISORDER

We will not delve deeply into the various diagnoses or their treatments since we are more concerned with access to care and cost. There are currently two widely established systems that classify mental disorders—*ICD-10 Chapter V: Mental and Behavioural disorders*, since 1949 part of the International Classification of Diseases produced by the WHO, and the *Diagnostic and Statistical Manual of Mental Disorders* produced by the American Psychiatric Association since 1952. Other classifications may be used in non-western countries, such as *Chinese Classification of Mental Disorders and* other manuals may be used by those of alternative theoretical persuasions for example the *Psychodynamic Diagnostic Manual.* Children have a range of disorders for example *autism, spectrum disorders, oppositional defiant disorder, conduct disorder, and attention deficit hyper activity disorder which* may continue into adulthood. Some disorders are chronic and some are transient. For example around half of people initially diagnosed with Bipolar disorder achieve syndromal recovery. Internationally, people report equal or greater disability from commonly occurring mental conditions than from commonly occurring physical conditions. The proportion with access to professional help for mental disorders is far lower, however, even among those assessed as having a severely disabling condition. In terms of total disability—adjusted life years which is an estimate of how many years of life are lost due to premature death or to being in a state of poor health and disability, mental disorders rank amongst the most disabling conditions. Unipolar depressive disorder is the third leading cause of disability worldwide. Among the other disorders that contribute inordinately to disability worldwide we must mention schizophrenia, alcohol-use, drug-use, bipolar disorder, panic disorder, primary insomnia and post-traumatic disorder. The diagnosis and treatment is beyond the scope of this book but needless to say the management of a mental disorder or even more than one disorder in a single patient can be complex and require special pharmacy and perhaps special institutions. The extent of this type of problem not only in this country but also in the world requires expensive Pharma, trained personnel as well as institutions. Management involves psychiatrists, psychologists, psychiatric nursing, psychotherapists, counselors, and public health professionals. Therapy may involve psychotherapy, psychoanalysis, medications, and even electroconvulsive therapy. Prevention has been tried as an effective way of reducing the disease burden and has been used as a means of saving public expenditure.

Mental disorders are common. Worldwide more than one in three people in most countries report sufficient criteria for at least one at some point in their lives. In the United States 46% qualify for a mental illness at some point. Anxiety disorders are the most common in all but one country followed by mood disorders in all but two countries while substance disorders and impulse-control disorders were consistently less prevalent. A 2004 cross-Europe study found that approximately one-in-four people reported meeting criteria at some point in their lives for at least one of the DSM-IV disorders assessed. Approximately 7% of a preschool pediatric sample were given a psychiatric diagnosis in one clinical study, and approximately 105 of 1-and 2 year olds were assessed as having significant emotional/ behavioral problems based on parent and pediatrician reports. Each year73 million women are afflicted with major depression and suicide is ranked 7th as a cause of death for women. The prevalence of mental disorders in the American and European societies leads to significant cost and economic strain for the medical care systems and for the training programs that must be supported.

DENTAL CARE

It must be recognized that dental care is a very important part of total health care. The usual insurance policy that is purchased or provided by the employer does not include dental care and as a result it is often disregarded as important and dental care and problems are often ignored when times are hard and money is tight. Small problems quickly become big problems that require expensive restorations, surgery, or even total replacement all of which may have been avoidable with routine care or early recognition. This is especially important in children. Besides care of teeth the routine exam is important for the diagnosis of oral cancer, gum disease, tongue problems, head and neck cancer, and other problems associated with diabetes, HIV/AIDS, heart disease, methamphetamine, and temporo-mandibular joint problems. A root-canal procedure at $1500 or $1600 will generate appreciation for dental coverage.

PHYSIOTHERAPY: There has been an increased emphasis on physiotherapy in recent years. Much of the emphasis came with the insurance companies as a way of getting patients out of the hospital sooner. This led to the establishment of physiotherapy hospitals that allowed the early transfer of postoperative patients after an operation where the daily charge per day was less because there was less staff. Physical therapy, often abbreviated PT is traditionally concerned with the remediation of impairments and disabilities more than postoperative recovery. One of the great disadvantages of being transferred to a PT hospital or institution immediately after surgery is that the surgeon or responsible doctor does not make daily rounds and releases responsibility to the nurses, physiotherapists and hired physicians on call. For those not requiring hospitalization physical therapy is usually performed in a clinic that is equipped for a variety of therapeutic exercises under the direction of a physical therapist or a physical therapist assistant. Besides the history and physical diagnosis and a physicians diagnosis and instructions, the therapist may use electrodiagnostic testing or electric stimulation. PTs practice in many settings: outpatient clinics, or offices, health and wellness clinics inpatient rehabilitation facilities, skilled nursing facilities, extended care facilities, private homes, education and research centers, schools, hospices, industrial and occupational environments and fitness and sports training facilities. Physical therapists also practice in non-patient care roles such as health policy and health insurance. Education qualifications vary greatly by country and may vary from having little formal education to having doctoral degrees, and post doctoral residencies. Some PTs specialize in specific clinical areas. The American Board of Physical Therapy Specialties lists eight specialist certifications: Cardiovascular& Pulmonary, Clinical Electrophysiology,

Geriatric, Integumentary, Neurological, Orthopedic, Pediatric, Sports, and Women's Health. Remuneration is relatively poor considering the level of training and the high standards.

PROSTHESES

In medicine the prosthesis or the prosthetic limb is an artificial device extension that replaces a missing body part. In the last 60 years we have witnessed the development of a host of artificial body parts that make life possible, or at times arm or leg function possible. We now have artificial hearts and lungs usually used on a temporary basis until a heart or lung transplant becomes available; there are artificial kidneys and livers on a temporary basis; we have prostheses to replace part or all of a leg or arm; and there are prosthetic heart valves, prosthetic arteries or veins, prosthetic parts for the skull or abdomen, and prostheses for reconstruction of a jaw or a face and even artificial or laboratory skin. These are obviously an important part of medical care for the patient and marvelous techniques for the surgeon and absolutely important for the patient suffering traumatic injuries such as the soldier or radical surgery such as some cancer patients or extensive burns. Some of these prostheses are very expensive and may not always be covered by insurance. The surgeries may be multiple and the hospitalizations long not to mention rehabilitation and long-term care. Again while these exist they may not be available to all. Other prosthetic devices that are often required as part of life but not necessarily available to all are eye glasses and hearing aids and dentures. Ideally under a system of universal coverage for health care they will be available on the basis of need. For completeness we should mention orthotics for foot and ankle injuries, pain, and discomfort. Special shoes and braces are available for such conditions.

NURSING HOME

As we come *to* the end of our dissertation on medical care it is appropriate to give some thought to the establishment we call The Nursing Home. It is where many of us will spend the end of life not always by choice and many times by necessity. The reasons for being settled in a nursing home can vary from physical disability, to mental decline, to inability to manage with safety or competence or because you are comatose or maybe just because your children or relatives or friends have decided with or without your permission that this the only proper or satisfactory solution. There is almost always a mental or physical problem that the patient or family or doctor cannot handle any more. A nursing home, convalescent home, skilled nursing unit, rest home, intermediate care, or old folks home (all variations of the nursing home) provide care and residence for people who require constant nursing care and have significant deficiencies with activities of daily living. Residents include the elderly and younger adults with physical or mental disabilities. Residents in a skilled nursing facility may also receive physical, occupational, and other rehabilitative therapies following an accident or illness. In the United States, a skilled nursing facility is a nursing home certified to participate in, and be reimbursed by Medicare. Medicare is the federal program primarily for the aged who contributed to Social Security and Medicare while they were employed. A "Nursing Facility" or "NF" is a nursing home certified to participate in and be reimbursed by Medicaid. Medicaid is the federal program implemented with each state to provide health care and related services to those who are "poor". Each state defines poverty and therefore eligibility. Those eligible for Medicaid may be aged, disabled, or children(e.g. Children's Health Insurance Programs-CHIPS and Maternal-Child wellness and food programs).

Each state licenses its nursing homes making them subject to the state's laws and regulations. Nursing Homes may chose to participate in Medicare and/or Medicaid. If they pass a survey (inspection) they are 'certified' and are also subject to federal regulations. All or part of a nursing home may participate in Medicare and/or Medicaid. In the United States nursing Homes which participate in Medicare and/or Medicaid are required to have licensed practical nurses on duty 24 hours a day. For at least 8 Hours per day, 7 days per week there must be a registered nurse on duty. Nursing homes are managed by a licensed Nursing Home Administrator. Unlike US nursing there is no standardized training or licensing requirements for nursing home administrators, though most states require a federal license and many states such as California have their own licensure for administrators. In 2005 there were 16,516 nursing homes in the United States. There are states that have other levels of care offered to elderly and other adults who are able to live in the community. For instance, Connecticut has Residential Care Homes that are licensed by the State Department of Public Health and provide 24-hour supervision in a home-like atmosphere.

SERVICES: Services provided in a nursing home include services of nurses, nursing aides, and assistants; physical, occupational, and speech therapy; social workers and recreational assistants and room and board. They also provide transportation. Most care is provided by CNAs (certified nursing assistants). In 2004 there were on average 40 certified nursing assistants per 100 resident beds. The number of registered nurses and licensed practical nurses were significantly lower at 7per resident beds and 13 per resident beds respectively. Medicare covers nursing home care for up to 100days for beneficiaries who require skilled nursing care or rehabilitation services following an hospitalization of at least 3 hospital days. The program does not cover nursing care if only custodial care is needed. To be eligible for Medicare-covered skilled nursing facility care a physician must certify that the beneficiary needs daily skilled nursing care or other skilled rehabilitation services that are related to the hospitalization and that these services can be provided only on an inpatient basis. SNF services may be offered in a free-standing or hospital based facility. A free-standing facility is generally part of a nursing home that covers Medicare SNF services as well as long-term care services for people who pay out-of-pocket, through Medicaid or through a long-term-care insurance policy. Generally Medicare patients make up just a small portion of the total resident population of a free-standing nursing home. Medicaid also covers nursing home care for certain persons who require custodial care, meet a states means—tested income and assets tests and require a level of care offered in a nursing home. Nursing home residents have physical or cognitive impairments and require 24-hour care.

The cost of staying in a nursing home can be equal to several thousand dollars per month or more. In fact cheaper nursing homes cost about $45,000 a year, whereas the most expensive ones can cost up to $ 200,000 per year. Some deplete their resources on the high cost of care. If eligible, Medicaid will cover continued stays in nursing homes for these individuals for life. However they require that the patient be "spent down" to a low asset level first by either depleting their life savings or asset-protecting them often using an elder law attorney.

NURSING HOMES IN THE UNITED KINGDOM

Have similarities to those in the United States. One similarity is they all cost money and are expensive. In 2002 nursing homes became known as care homes with nursing, and residential homes became known as care homes. These are all regulated by different organizations in England, Scotland Wales, and North Ireland. To enter a care home you need an assessment of needs and of your financial condition from your local council. You may also have an assessment by a nurse should you require nursing care. The cost of a care home is means tested in England. As of April 2009 in England, the lower capital limit is 13,500 pounds. At this level all income from pensions, savings, benefits and other sources, except a personal expense allowance (currently 21.90 pounds) will go to paying the care home fees. The local council pays the remaining contribution provided the room occupied is not more expensive than the local council's normal rate currently 364.48 pounds for Hampshire for example. If the resident is paying more than this the council will not pay anything and contributions from a third party or from charity must be found or the resident move to a cheaper care home. Between the lower and the upper capital limits, the resident pays their income less personal expenses allowance + 1 pound per week for every 250 pounds capital between lower and higher limit. The council pays the rest, subject to the same conditions as before. It is therefore preferable to find a home within the councils limit if council's funding is likely to be required to avoid a forced move later. Patients with capital over more than 23,000 pounds pay the full cost of the care home, until the total value of their assets fall below the threshold. Patients who require additional nursing care are assessed for this and receive additional support through the National Health Service; this is known as Funded Nursing Care. The NHS has full responsibility for funding the whole placement if the resident in a care home with nursing meets the criteria for NHS continuing health care. This identified by a multi-disciplinary assessment process as detailed on DOH website. Care homes for adults in England are regulated by Care Quality Commission for Social Care Inspection, and each care home is inspected at least every three years. In Wales the Care Standards Inspectorate for Wales has responsibility for oversight. In Scotland Social Care and Social Work Improvement Scotland otherwise known as th the Care Inspectorate, and in Northern Ireland the Regulation and Quality Improvement Authority in Northern Ireland.

QUEBEC: Long term care facilities exist under three types, public, subsidized, and private. Public and subsidized differ only in their ownership, all other aspects of funding, admission criteria, cost to the individuals are all regulated by the Quebec Ministry of Health and Social Services. Private facilities are completely independent from government ownership and funding and have their own admission criteria. They must maintain certain provincial standards and require licensing from the ministry.

MEDICAL PRODUCTS, RESEARCH AND DEVELOPMENT

The Food and Drug Administration (FDA) is the primary institution tasked with the safety and effectiveness of human and veterinary drugs. It is also responsible for making sure drug information is accurately and informatively presented to the public. The FDA approves products and establishes drug labeling, drug standards and medical device manufacturing standards. It sets performance standards for radiation and ultrasonic equipment. One of the more contentious issues related to drug safety is immunity from prosecution. In 2004 the FDA reversed a federal policy, arguing that FDA premarket approval overrides most claims for damages under state law for medical devices. In 2008 this was confirmed by the Supreme Court in Riegel v. Medtronic. On 30 June 2006, an FDA ruling went into effect extending protection from lawsuits to pharmaceutical manufacturers, even if it was found that they submitted fraudulent clinical trial data to the FDA in their quest for approval. This left consumers who experience serious health consequences from drug use little recourse. In 2007, opposition was raised in the Congressional House to the FDA ruling but the Senate upheld the ruling. On 4 March 2009, an important Supreme Court decision was handed down. In Wyeth vs Levine the court asserted that state-level rights of action could not be pre-empted by federal immunity and could provide "appropriate relief for injured consumers" In June 2009, under the Public Readiness and Emergency Preparedness Act, Secretary of Health and human Services Kathleen Sibelius signed an order extending protection to vaccine makers and federal officials from prosecution during a declared health emergency related to the administration of the swine flu vaccine.

As in most other countries, the manufacture and production of pharmaceuticals and medical devices is carried out by private companies. The research and development of medical devices and pharmaceuticals is supported by both public and private sources of funding. In 2003 research and development expenditures were approximately $95 billion with $40billion coming from public sources and $55 billion coming from private sources. These investments into medical research have made the United States the leader in medical innovation, measured either in terms of revenue or the number of new drugs and devices introduced. In 2006, the United States accounted for three quarters of the worlds biotechnology revenues and 82% of the world's R&D spending in biotechnology. According to multiple international pharmaceutical trade groups, the high cost of patented drugs in the U.S. has encouraged substantial reinvestment in such research and development.

The drug companies in the US do have political clout. The United States is one of the two countries in the world that allows direct-to-consumer advertising of prescription drugs. Critics note that drug ads cost money which they believe have raised the overall price of drugs. When health care legislation was being written in 2009, the drug companies were asked to support the legislation in return for not allowing importation of drugs from foreign countries. During the 1990s, the price of prescription drugs became a major issue in American politics as the prices of many new drugs increased exponentially, and many citizens discovered that neither the government nor their insurer would cover the cost of such drugs. Per capita the U.S. spends more on pharmaceuticals than any other country. National expenditures on pharmaceuticals accounted for 12.9 % of total health care costs. Some 25% of out-of-pocket spending by individuals is for prescription drugs. The U.S. government has taken the position that the U.S. drug prices are rising because U.S. consumers are effectively subsidizing costs which drug companies cannot recover from consumers in other countries(because many other countries use their bulk purchasing power to aggressively negotiate drug prices.) Currently, U.S. as a purchaser of pharmaceuticals negotiates some drug prices but is forbidden by law to negotiate drug prices for the Medicare Program due to the Medicare prescription Drug, Improvement, and Modernization Act passed in 2003. Democrats have charged that the purpose of this provision is merely to allow the pharmaceutical industry to profiteer off of the Medicare program. Perhaps this a good point to mention statistics relating to harmful drug reactions. National statistics reveal that bad drug reactions send 700,000 people to the emergency room annually. Accidental overdoses and allergic reactions to prescription drugs were the most frequent cause of serious illness according to the study. People over 65 faced the greatest risk. These involved some of the most widely used medicines such as insulin and antibiotics. This may be an underestimate since drug reactions are often misdiagnosed. The study found that a small group of commonly used drugs were implicated such as insulin, warfarin, and amoxicillin. The results for 2004-05 were published in the Journal of the American Medical Association. The CDC has estimated that about 130 million Americans use prescribed medication every month. U.S. consumers buy far more medicine per person than anywhere else in the world.

HEALTHCARE SPENDING AND THE HEALTHCARE DEBATE

Now that we have outlined most of the parameters that comprise Health Care, It quickly becomes obvious that health care is not only complex but it is also very expensive even in a very rich nation. But how rich do you have to be to afford total health care on a personal or on a national level. Current estimates put U.S. health care spending at approximately 16% of GDP or over $2.26 trillion, or $7,439 per person, up from $2.1 trillion or $7,026 per capita the previous year. Growth in spending is projected to average 6.7% annually over the period 2007 through 2017. In 2009, the United States, federal, state and local governments, corporations, and individuals together spent $2.5trillion, or $8,047 per person on health care. This amount represented 17.3% of the GDP, up from 16.2% in2008. Health insurance costs are rising faster than wages or inflation and medical causes were cited by about half of bankruptcy filers in the United States in 2001. The Congressional Budget Office has found that about half of all growth in healthcare spending in the past several decades was associated with changes in medical care made possible by advances in technology. Other factors include higher income, changes in insurance coverage, and rising prices. Hospitals and physician spending take the largest share of the health care dollar, while prescription drugs take about 10%. Prices paid for health care services are much higher in the U.S. While the U.S. spends more than other countries in the Organization for Economic Co-operation and Development, the use of healthcare services in the US is below the OECD median by most measures. Economist Hans Sennholz has argued that the Medicare and Medicaid programs may be the main reasons for the rising healthcare costs.

Health care spending in the United States is concentrated in the top 1% of the population which accounted for 27% of aggregate healthcare spending.

Seniors spend, on average far more on health care costs than either working age adults or children. The 2008 edition of the Dartmouth Atlas of Health Care found that providing Medicare beneficiaries with severe chronic diseases with more intense health care in the last two years of life is not associated with better outcomes. Acute hospital care accounts for over half of the spending for Medicare beneficiaries in the last two years of life. In September 2008 *the Wall Street Journal* reported that consumers were reducing their health care spending in response to the current economic slowdown.

HEALTH CARE PAYMENT: BUNDLED PAYMENT; CAPITATION (HEALTHCARE); AND FEE-FOR-SERVICE

Doctors and hospitals are generally funded by payments from patients and insurance plans in return for services rendered (fee-for-service or FFS). Around 84.7% of Americans have some form of health insurance.; either through their employer or the employer of their spouse or parent, purchased individually (8.9%) or provided by government programs(27.8%); (there is some overlap in these figures). All government health care programs have restricted eligibility, and there is no government health insurance company which covers all Americans. Americans without health insurance in2007 totaled 15.3%of the population, or 45.7 million people. Among those whose employer pays for health insurance, the employee may be required to contribute part of the cost, while the employer chooses the insurance company and for large groups, negotiates with the insurance company. In 2004, private insurance paid for 36% of personal health expenditures, private out-of-pocket 15%, federal government 34%, state and local governments 11%, and other private funds 4%. Due to a "dishonest and in-efficient system" that sometimes inflates bills to ten times the actual cost, even insured patients can be billed more than the real cost of their care. Insurance for dental and vision care (except for visits to the ophthalmologist, which are covered by regular health insurance) is usually sold separately. Prescription drugs are usally handled separately from medical services though not by government services

Individuals with private or government insurance are limited to medical facilities which accept the particular type of medical insurance they carry. Visits to facilities outside the insurance company's network are usually either not covered or the patient must bear more of the cost. Hospitals negotiate with insurance programs to set reimbursement rates; some rates for government insurance programs are set by law. The sum paid to a doctor for a service rendered to an insured patient is generally less than that paid out-of-pocket by an uninsured patient. In return for this discount the insurance company includes the doctor as part of their network. The negotiated rate may not cover the cost of the service, but providers (doctors and hospitals) can refuse to accept a given type of insurance, including Medicare and Medicaid. Low reimbursement rates have generated complaints from providers, and some patients with government and even private insurance have difficulty finding nearby providers for certain types of medical services.

Charity care for those who cannot pay is sometimes available and is usually funded by non-profit foundations, religious orders, government subsidies or services donated by employees. Perhaps the most common charity is given by the doctor or surgeon who never gets paid for his/her services. Massachusetts and New Jersey have programs where the state will pay for health care when the patient cannot afford to. The city and county of San Francisco is also implementing a citywide health care program for all uninsured residents, limited to those whose incomes and net worth are below an eligibility threshold. Some cities and counties operate or provide subsidies to private facilities open to all regardless of the ability to pay but even here patients who can afford to pay or who have insurance are generally charged.

The Emergency Medical Treatment and Active labor Act requires virtually all hospitals to accept all patients regardless of the ability to pay for emergency room care. The Act does not provide access to non-emergency room care for patients who cannot afford to pay for health care nor does it provide the benefit of preventive care and the continuity of a primary care physician. Emergency care is generally more expensive than an urgent care clinic or a doctor's office visit especially if a condition has worsened due to putting off needed care. Emergency rooms are typically at or near over capacity. Long wait times have become a problem nationally, and in urban areas some ERs are put on "diversion" on a regular basis, meaning that ambulances are directed to take patients elsewhere.

PRIVATE INSURANCE AND HEALTH CARE

Most Ameicans under age 65 (59.3%) receive their health insurance coverage through an employer (which includes both private and public sector employers) under group coverage although this percentage is declining. Costs for employer-paid health insurance are rising rapidly: since 2001 premiums for family coverage have increased 78%, while wages have risen 19% and inflation has risen 17%, according to a study by the Kaiser Family Foundation. Workers with employer-sponsored insurance also contribute; in 2007 the average premium paid by covered workers is 16% for single coverage and 28% for family coverage. In addition to their premium contributions, most covered workers face additional payments when they use health care services, in the form of deductibles and copayments.

Just less than 9% of the population purchases individual health care insurance. Insurance payments are a form of cost sharing, this cost sharing mechanism picks up much of the cost of health care but individuals must often pay up-front a deductible or a copayment which is a small part of the cost of every procedure. Private insurance accounts for 35% of the total health spending in the United States, by far the largest share of the cost among OECD countries. Besides the United States, Canada and France are the other two countries where private insurance represents more than 10% of total health spending. Provider networks can be used to reduce costs by negotiating favorable fees, or selecting cost effective providers but providers are limited also by the necessity of making a living and paying overhead just like any business. A survey in 2009 by America's Health Insurance Plans found that patients going to out of network providers are sometimes charged extremely high fees. PPOs which are more loosely managed as far as having to obtain care within "network' have edged out HMOs and the HMOs have evolved towards less tightly managed models. The HMO refers to a Health Maintenance Organization and the original models such as Kaiser Permanente in Oakland California and The Health Insurance Plan(HIP) in New York were staff models which owned their own facilities and employed the doctors and other health care professionals who staffed them. The idea of an HMO was not to merely treat disease but to maintain health and practice preventive health care. They developed and disseminated guidelines for cost-effective care. Despite all this they have steadily lost market share to the more loosely managed PPOs and loosely managed networks of providers with whom health plans have negotiated discounted fees. It is common today for a physician or hospital to have contracts with a dozen or more health plans each with different referral networks, contracts with different diagnostic facilities, and different practice guidelines.

GOVERNMENT PROGRAMS

Government programs directly cover 27.8%of the population(83 million) including the elderly, disabled, children, veterans, some of the poor, and the military both active and retirees. Public spending accounts for between 45% and 56% of U.S. health care spending. Per capita spending on health care by the U.S. government placed it among the top 10 highest spenders among United Nations member countries in 2004.

Government funded programs include:

- Medicare, generally covering citizens 65 years and older and the disabled.
- Medicaid, generally covering low income people, children, pregnant women and the disabled
- State Children's health insurance program for low income children
- Various programs for federal employees, including TRICARE for military personnel
- The Veterans Administration which provides care to veterans
- Title X which funds reproductive health care
- State and local health department clinic
- Indian health service
- National Institutes of health treat patients who enroll in research for free
- Medical Corps of various branches of the military
- Certain county and state hospitals
- Government run community clinics

The exemption of employer-sponsored health benefits from income tax distorts the health care market. The value of this lost tax revenue amounts to $150 billion a year. People who buy insurance in the individual market must pay for premiums with after-tax money. As a result of this 65% of the non-elderly population receives health insurance at the workplace. In addition to this the government allows full tax shelter at the highest marginal rate to investors in health savings account. Some have argued that this tax incentive does little for the national health care because the most wealthy in the society tend to be the most healthy. HSAs segregate insurance pools into those for the wealthy and those for the less wealthy and thereby makes insurance cheaper for the rich. However the HAS accounts can only be used towards HAS qualified expenses such as doctor fees and cannot be used for expenses like cosmetic surgery. There are also state and local programs for the poor. In 2007, Medicaid provided health care coverage for 40 million low-income Americans and Medicare provided health care coverage for 41.4 million elderly and disabled Americans. Enrollment in Medicare is expected to reach 77 million by 2031 when the baby-boom generation is fully enrolled. The number of physicians accepting Medicaid has decreased in recent years due to relatively high administrative costs and low reimbursements. In 1997 the federal government also created the State Children's Health Insurance Program (SCHIP), a joint federal-state program to insure children in families that earn too much to qualify for Medicaid but cannot afford health insurance. SCHIP covered 6.6 million children in 2006, but the program is already facing shortfalls in many states. The government has also mandated access to emergency care regardless of insurance through the Emergency Medical Treatment and Labor Act (EMTALA) passed in 1986, but EMTALA is an unfunded mandate.

The Uninsured

Some Americans just do not qualify for health insurance coverage under any form due to lack of employment, money, desire, and government programs. In some cases charity fills the need if no free program is available they go without needed medical care. According to the U.S. Census Bureau, in 2007, 45.7 million people in the U.S. were without health insurance for at least part of the year. Other studies have placed the number of uninsured in the years 2007-2008 as high as 86.7 million, about 29%of the population.

A 2003 study in *Health Affairs* estimated that uninsured people in the U.S. received approximately $35 billion in uncompensated care in 2001. The study noted that the amount per capita was about half what the average insured person received. The study found that various levels of government finance most uncompensated care. The role of government in the health care market is huge. Numerous publicly funded health care programs help to provide for the elderly, disabled military service families and veterans, children and the poor. Federal law ensures access to emergency services regardless of ability to pay however universal care has not been implemented. The amount of money that the U.S. spends would, in other countries, cover the entire population. The U.S. as a matter of oft-stated policy does not regulate prices of services from private providers, assuming the private sector to do it better. Massachusetts has adopted a universal health care system through the Massachusetts 2006 Health Reform Statute. It mandates that all residents who can afford to do so purchase health insurance, and provides subsidized insurance plans so nearly everyone can afford health insurance. Cost of health care has risen faster than predicted. In July 2009, Connecticut passed into law a plan called SustiNet. with the Goal of achieving health-care coverage of 98%of its residents by 2014.

Healthcare Regulation and Oversight

Healthcare is subject to extensive regulation at both the federal and state levels. Under this system the federal government cedes primary responsibility to the states under the McCarran-Ferguson Act. Essential regulation includes the licensure of health care providers at the state level and testing and approval of pharmaceuticals and medical devices by the Food and Drug Administration and laboratory testing. States regulate the health insurance market. Although the states may mandate certain procedures be covered by the insurance companies there are exceptions that such mandates do not apply to the self-funded health care plans offered by large employers. In 2010 the Patient Protection and Affordable Care Act was passed which contains a mandate requiring all citizens to purchase health insurance. This mandate as well as the law has been reviewed by the Supreme Court.

At the federal level, the United States Department of Health and Human Services oversees the various federal agencies involved in health care. These are part of the United States Public Health Service and include the Food and Drug Administration, the Centers for Disease Prevention, the Agency of Health Care Research and Quality, the Agency for Toxic Substances and Disease Registry, and the National Institutes of Health. State governments maintain state health departments and local governments often have their own departments, usually branches of the state health department. Regulations of a state board may have executive and police strength to enforce state health laws. The McCarran-Ferguson Act, which cedes regulation to the states does not itself regulate insurance, nor does it mandate that states regulate insurance. "Acts of Congress" that do not purportedly regulate the "business of insurance" will not preempt state laws regulations that regulate the "business of insurance". Self-policing of providers by providers is a major part of oversight. Many health care organizations voluntarily submit to inspection and certification by the Joint Commission on Accreditation of Hospital Organizations, JCAHO. Providers also undergo testing to obtain board certification attesting to their skills. The Centers for Medicare and Medicaid Services (CMS) publishes an online searchable database of performance data on nursing homes

The Certificate of Need programs for cardiac care instituted in 1978 have not been found as effective programs to reduce costs and have not been renewed by most states and institutions after the federal requirement expired in 1986. The licensing of providers and privileges attending a license vary by state and even by the specialty Boards. Renewal may require evidence of credits for attendance at educational meetings or courses of training. In 1995, 36 states banned or restricted midwifery even though they have demonstrated equally safe deliveries to that of doctors. Moreover, psychologists, nurses, and pharmacologists are not allowed to prescribe medicines and nurses were not allowed to vaccinate without direct supervision. These restrictions limit care and reduce the availability of trained personnel to provide care. Many of these restrictions were lobbied for by the AMA. The American Medical Association also lobbied the government to limit the number of doctors since 1910, even though it is recognized now that the country faces a doctor shortage in the coming decades. It is also clear now that nurse practitioners and physician assistants will be necessary to fill the ranks of providers in offices, hospitals, operating rooms, emergency rooms, nursing homes, clinics and on the battlefield.

Effectiveness Compared to Other Countries

The CIA World Factbook ranked the United States 41st in the world for infant mortality and 46th for total life expectancy. Recent studies find growing gaps in life expectancy based on income and geography. In 2008, a government study found that life expectancy declined from 1983 to1999 for women in 180 counties and for men in180 counties with most of the life expectancy declines occurring in the Deep South. The gap is growing between rich and poor and by educational level but narrowing between men and women and by race. Obesity in the U.S. is the worst in the world and has been increasing. In an analysis of breast cancer, colorectal cancer and prostate cancer diagnosed during 1990-1994 in 31 countries, the United States had the highest five-year relative survival rate for breast cancer and prostate cancer, although survival was systematically and substantially lower in black U.S. men and women. There is a great deal of skepticism about the WHO analyses of efficiency, quality and satisfaction and not much to be gained by their rankings.

The costs of treating the uninsured must often be absorbed by providers such as charity, passed on to the insured via cost shifting and higher health insurance premiums or paid by taxpayers through higher taxes. However, hospitals and other providers are reimbursed for the cost of providing uncompensated care via a federal matching fund program. Each state enacts legislation governing the reimbursement of funds to providers. In Missouri, for example providers assessments totaling 800 million are matched—$2 for each assessed $1—to create a pool of approximately $2billion. By federal law these funds are transferred to the Missouri Hospital Association for disbursement to hospitals for the costs incurred providing uncompensated care including Disproportionate Share Payments (to hospitals with high quantities of uninsured patients.), Medicaid shortfalls, Medicaid Managed

Care payments to insurance companies and other cost incurred by hospitals. In New Hampshire, by statute, reimbursable uncompensated care costs shall include: charity care costs, any portion of Medicaid patient care costs that are unreimbursed by Medicaid payments and any portion of bad debt costs that the commissioner determines would meet the criteria under 42 U.S.C. section 1396-4(g) governing hospital specific limits on disproportionate share hospital payments under Title XIX of the Social Security Act.

A report published by the Kaiser Family Foundation in April 2008 found that economic downturns place a significant strain on state Medicaid and SCHIP programs. The authors estimated that a 1% increase in the unemployment rate would increase Medicaid and SCHIP enrollment by 1 million and increase the number of uninsured by 1.1 million. State spending on Medicaid and SCHIP would increase by $1.4 billion(total spending on these programs would increase by $3.4 billion) This increase would occur at the same time state government revenues were declining. During the last downturn the Jobs and Growth Tax Relief Reconciliation Act of 2003 included federal assistance to states which helped states avoid tightening their Medicaid and SCHIP eligibility rules.

ADMINISTRATIVE COSTS

The health care system in the U.S. has a vast number of players. There are hundreds if not thousands of insurance companies in the U.S. This system has considerable administrative overhead, far greater than in nationalized, single-payer systems, such as Canada's. An oft-cited study by Harvard Medical School and the Canadian Institute for health information determined that some 31% of U.S. health care dollars or more than $1,000 per person per year, went to health care administrative costs, nearly double the administrative overhead in Canada, [on a percentage basis] According to the insurance industry group America's Health Insurance Plans, administrative costs for private health insurance plans have averaged approximately 12% of premiums over the last 40 years. There has been a shift in the type and distribution of administrative expenses over that period. The cost of adjudicating claims has fallen, while insurers are spending more time on other administrative activities such as medical management, nurse help lines, and negotiating discounted fees with health care providers. A 2003 study published by Blue Cross and Blue Shield Association also found that health insurer administrative costs were approximately 11% to 12% of premiums with BC and BS reporting slightly lower administrative costs, on average than commercial insurers. The largest increases in administrative costs were in customer service and information technology and the largest decreases were in provider services and contracting. The McKinsey Global institute estimated that excess spending on "health administration and insurance" accounted for as much as 21% of the estimated total excess spending.($477 billion in 2003).

COVERAGE

Enrollment rules in private and governmental programs result in millions of Americans going without health care coverage, including children. The U.S. Census Bureau estimated that 45.7 million Americans (15.3% of the total population) had no health insurance coverage in 2007. The Census Bureau writes that "health insurance coverage is likely to be underreported ". Studies have shown approximately one third of this 45.7 million person population of uninsured is actually eligible for government insurance programs such as Medicare/Medicaid, but has elected not to enroll. The largest proportion of the uninsured is persons earning in excess of 50,000 dollars per annum, with those earning over 70,000 dollars comprising the fastest growing segment of the uninsured population. U.S. citizens who earn too much money to qualify for government assistance with insurance programs but who do not earn enough to purchase a private insurance plan make up approximately 2.7%of the total U.S. population.(8.2 million). Some states(like California) do offer insurance coverage for children of low income families but not for adults; other states do not offer such coverage at all. Although EMTALA keeps alive many working class people who are badly injured the 1986 law neither requires the provision of preventive or rehabilitative care, nor subsidizes such care and it does nothing about the difficulties in the American mental health system.

Coverage gaps also occur among the insured population. An even bigger problem is the under insured, and the most credible estimate of the number of people in the United States who have died because of lack of medical care was provided by a study carried out by Harvard Medical School Professors Himmelstein and Woolhandler (*New England Journal of Medicine 336, no11, 1997*). They concluded that almost 100,000people died in the United States each year because of lack of needed care. Another study by the Commonwealth Fund published in *Health Affairs* estimated 16 million U.S. adults were underinsured in 2003. The study defined under insurance as characterized by at least one of the following conditions: annual out-of-pocket medical expenses totaling 10% or more of income or 5% or more among adults with incomes below 200% of the poverty level; or health plan deductibles equaling or exceeding 5% of income. The underinsured were more likely than those with adequate insurance to forgo health care, report financial stress because of medical bills and experience coverage gaps for such items as prescription drugs. The study found that underinsurance disproportionately affects those with lower incomes—73% of the underinsured in the study population had annual incomes below 200% of the federal poverty level. Another study focusing on the effects of being underinsured found that individuals with private insurance were less likely to be diagnosed with late stage cancer than either the uninsured or Medicaid beneficiaries. Coverage gaps and affordability also surfaced in a 2007 international comparison by the Commonwealth Fund. Among adults surveyed in the U.S., 37% reported that they had foregone needed medical care in the previous year because of cost; either skipping medications, avoiding seeing a doctor when sick, or avoiding other recommended care. The rate was even higher—42%—among those with chronic conditions. The study reported that these rates were well above those found in the other six countries surveyed: Australia, Canada, Germany, the Netherlands, New Zealand, and the UK.

Mental Health

A lack of mental health coverage for Americans bears significant ramifications for the US economy and social system because a report (US surgeon General).found that mental illnesses are the second leading cause of disability in the country and it affects 20% of Americans. It is estimated that less than half of all people with mental illnesses receive treatment due to factors such as stigma and lack of access to care. The Paul Wellstone mental Health and Addiction Equity Act of 2008 mandates that group health plans provide mental health and substance-related disorder benefits that are at least equivalent to benefits offered for medical and surgical procedures. The legislation renews and expands provisions of the Mental Health Parity Act of 1996. This requires financial equity for annual and lifetime mental health benefits, and compels parity in treatment limits and expands all equity provisions to addiction services. Up to 2008 insurance companies used loopholes and, though providing financial equity they often worked around the laws by applying unequal co-payments or setting limits on the number of days spent in in-patient or out-patient treatment facilities.

Medical Underwriting and the Uninsurable

In most states in the U.S., people seeking to purchase health insurance directly must undergo medical underwriting. Insurance companies seeking to mitigate the problem of adverse selection and manage their risk pools screen applicants for pre-existing conditions. Insurers reject many applicants or quote increased rates for those with pre-existing conditions. Diseases that can make an individual uninsurable include serious conditions such as arthritis, cancer, and heart disease, but also such common ailments as acne, being 20 pounds overweight, and old sports injuries. An estimated 5 million of those without health insurance are considered uninsurable because of pre-existing conditions. Proponents of medical underwriting argue that it ensures that individual health insurance premiums are kept as low as possible. Critics of underwriting say that it prevents many people with relatively minor problems from ever obtaining health insurance.

One large industry survey found that 13% of applicants for individual health insurance who went through medical underwriting were denied coverage in 2004. Declination rates increased significantly with age, rising from 5% for those under 18 to just under 1/3 for those aged 60 to64. Among those who were offered coverage the study found that 76% received offers at standard premium rates, and 22%were offered higher rates. The frequency of increased premiums also increased with age so for applicants over 40, roughly half were affected by medical underwriting either in the form of denial or increased premiums. In contrast, almost 90% of applicants in their 20s were offered contracts and 3/4 of those were offered standard rates. A study by the commonwealth Fund in 2001 found that among those aged 19-64 who sought individual contracts during the previous three years the majority found it unaffordable. And less than a third ended up buying insurance. Some states have outlawed medical underwriting as a prerequisite for individually purchased health coverage. These states tend to have the highest premiums for individual health insurance.

DEMOGRAPHIC DIFFERENCES: HEALTH DISPARITIES AND RACE

In the United States health disparities are well documented in ethnic minorities such as African Americans, Native Americans and Hispanics. When compared to whites, these minority groups have higher incidence of chronic diseases, higher mortality, and poorer health outcomes. Among the disease specific examples of racial and ethnic disparities in the United States is the cancer incidence rate among African Americans, which is 25% higher than among whites. In addition, adult African Americans and Hispanics have approximately twice the risk as whites of developing diabetes. Minorities also have higher rates of cardiovascular disease, and HIV/AIDS than whites. Caucasian Americans have a much lower life expectancy than Asian Americans. Levels of education also affect life expectancy. Some inequalities are the result of income disparities since uninsured Americans are less likely to receive preventive services. For example minorities are less likely to be screened for colon cancer and the death rate for colon cancer has increased among African Americans and Hispanics.

Public spending for health care is highly correlated with age; average per capita public spending for seniors was more than five times that for children ($6,921 vs $1,225) Average public spending for non-Hispanic blacks ($2,973) was slightly higher than that for whites ($2,675) while spending for Hispanics ($1,967) was significantly lower than the population average ($2,612). Seniors comprise 13% of the population but take 1/3 of all prescription drugs.

FOOD AND DRUG ADMINISTRATION

When Health Care Legislation was being written in2009, the drug companies were asked to support the legislation in return for not allowing importation of drugs from foreign countries.

During the 1990s the price of prescription drugs became a major issue in American politics as the prices of many new drugs increased exponentially, and many citizens discovered that neither the government nor their insurer would cover the cost of these drugs. Per capita the U.S. spends more on pharmaceuticals than any other country. National expenditures on pharmaceuticals accounted for 12.9% of total health care costs, compared to an OECD average of 17.7%. Some 25% of out-of-pocket spending by individuals is for prescription drugs. The cost of drugs is contentious because many other countries use their bulk purchasing power to aggressively negotiate drug prices. The US position(and that of the drug lobbying group) is that governments of such countries are free riding on the backs of U.S. consumers. Currently, the U.S. as a purchaser of pharmaceuticals negotiates some prices but is forbidden by law from negotiating drug prices for the Medicare program due to the Medicare Prescription Drug, Improvement and Modernization Act passed in 2003. Democrats charge that the purpose of this Act is to allow the pharmaceutical industry to profiteer off the Medicare program which is already in financial trouble.

THE HEALTH CARE DEBATE: IS THERE A BETTER SYSTEM? CAN WE AFFORD PPACA

This rather long examination of the world of heath care should provide us with a conclusion as to what the ideal system is or at least some strong opinions as to where we want to go, how we are going to get there and what can we really afford without destroying the economy. We probably all agree that health care, good heath care, easily accessible health care, and finally universal health care are absolutely essential for the present and the future of our country and our way of life. We are all aware of the great advancements that have occurred in medicine, surgery, and mental health in the last 75 years. The U.S. has been the stage where many if not most of the medical marvels in drugs, radiology, medical instrumentation, organ transplantation, heart surgery, ultrasound, cancer therapy, chemotherapy, and antibiotics and so many others have taken place. We can well be proud of our institutions, our medical complexes and medical schools and our vast research and development capabilities both private companies and government institutions like the National Institutes of Health or the CDC. With all this expertise and progressive energy surely we can design a system or at least analyze our present and plan for the future. The attempts to modify or change the system during the Clinton administration failed for many reasons, one of which was that congress didn't like or approve it. The new PPACA or Patient Protection and Affordable Care Act was signed into law by president Barack Obama on March 23, 2010. This has not been totally implemented and will be phased in until 2015. This plan is basically designed and operated by the health insurance companies and supplements the existing government sponsored and managed health care entities such as

Medicare, Medicaid, Social Security, Veterans Administration, Tricare, and the Military system of care. The PPACA or the new health plan has been reviewed by the Supreme Court particularly the "mandate to buy insurance". The result of this review of constitutionality will be an important landmark in the history of medical care in this country. This discourse will not end up with a plan for the United States nor a possible budget. That is too complicated for this author. It is possible however to speculate on the basis of past history. It is clear that this country is investing a large portion of its economic resources annually to support the present health care system and that amount or portion of GDP (15%-17% annually) has been increasing annually. The annual cost to the U.S. is now in excess of two trillion dollars a year and climbing. We are now spending over $7,000 per capita compared to about 50-60% of that in other industrialized countries. Can we continue this trend without having serious economic difficulties. We have outstanding professional resources, doctors, nurses and paraprofessionals that are the equal of any in the world, well staffed hospitals and medical schools but we do not have universal coverage. Health care is not available to everyone, only to those who are covered by government programs or employment programs, or can afford the premiums of private insurance which are usually unaffordable by the poor, unemployed and the young. There are still 45 to 50 million people without insurance or other means of obtaining health care when needed except for charitable institutions (or doctors) and EMTALA a law that allows all to seek emergency care at any emergency room. We continue with for-profit insurance companies as the primary health care coverage for those below 65 years old. The economics spelled out above do not favor survival of a for-profit system unless we have an unprecedented era of high prosperity and mandatory coverage for all. PPACA (Obamacare) maybe the answer we are all looking for but that is doubtful.

Health Care Reimbursement Accounts

www.ingramcontent.com/pod-product-compliance
Lightning Source LLC
Chambersburg PA
CBHW020735180526
45163CB00001B/245